[英国]乌塔·弗里思 著　刘光源 译

自闭症

牛津通识读本·

Autism

A Very Short Introduction

译林出版社

图书在版编目（CIP）数据

自闭症／（英）乌塔·弗里思（Uta Frith）著；刘光源译．
南京：译林出版社，2018.12（2023.9重印）
（牛津通识读本）
书名原文：Autism: A Very Short Introduction
ISBN 978-7-5447-7518-2

Ⅰ.①自… Ⅱ.①乌… ②刘… Ⅲ.①孤独症－防治
Ⅳ.①R749.4

中国版本图书馆 CIP 数据核字（2018）第 210287 号

著作权合同登记号　图字：10-2020-573 号

自闭症　［英国］乌塔·弗里思／著　刘光源／译

责任编辑　许　丹　何本国
装帧设计　景秋萍
校　　对　张　萍
责任印制　董　虎

原文出版　Oxford University Press, 2008
出版发行　译林出版社
地　　址　南京市湖南路 1 号 A 楼
邮　　箱　yilin@yilin.com
网　　址　www.yilin.com
市场热线　025-86633278
排　　版　南京展望文化发展有限公司
印　　刷　江苏凤凰通达印刷有限公司
开　　本　890 毫米 ×1260 毫米　1/32
印　　张　8.375
插　　页　4
版　　次　2018 年12月第 1 版
印　　次　2023 年9月第 5 次印刷
书　　号　ISBN 978-7-5447-7518-2
定　　价　39.00 元

序 言

魏坤琳

乌塔·弗里思是我们这个时代最伟大的自闭症研究者之一。在长达五十余年的研究生涯里面，她著作等身、贡献卓越，其理论和实践深远地影响了自闭症的科学研究。更难能可贵的是，她是一位充满同理心、对自闭症群体及其家庭有深刻理解的女性，为自闭症的科普做了大量的工作。而您手中这本书是她精心撰写的一本简约但全面、文字浅显但思想深刻的自闭症科普读物。

我的学术研究方向是认知心理学和认知神经科学，专长是人的感知运动控制。但是过去几年中，我开始有意识地涉及自闭症研究，因为我发现这是一个充满着未知和挑战、又被社会和广大自闭症家庭迫切需要的研究领域。美国目前的自闭症发病率约1/60；中国的官方数字尚缺，但粗略估计在1/100左右。考虑到中国的人口基数，我们的自闭症患者群体庞大，其影响了千万家庭的生活和幸福感，对社会保障、教育、医疗系统构成了严重的挑战。遗憾的是，目前科学家和医学界只揭开了自闭症的部分奥秘，也只提供了效果有限的干预手段。迄今为止，我们还没有直接、简单的医学诊断手段，而是主要依赖专业人员的临床观察和家长访谈；我们没有根除这种复杂的精神类疾病的行为学疗法，或者药物和基因疗法；我们甚至没有统一的认知和神经学理论来解释自闭症。

科研的滞后造成大众不能理解这些“来自星星的孩子”，也对如何有效地诊断、矫正和教育这些孩子感到疑惑。同时，市面上有成百上千的宣称能“治愈”自闭症的话术和骗术，有数不清的非科学、非专业的干预手段。甚至，某些研究者宣称自闭症是后天养育造成的，仅仅因为他们发现自闭症患儿和应激后创伤的患者之间存在行为特征的相似性。其实，这样的“理论”早已被自闭症的神经和心理学研究所推翻，因为大量科学证据表明自闭症是有基因基础伴随终身的神经发育障碍；环境对自闭症有影响，但不是致病的主因。可见，当科学还没解开所有谜团，伪科学和迷信总会有机会沉渣泛起。

乌塔·弗里思这本“牛津通识读本”的中文版出版得恰是时候。她从自闭症患者的故事入手，从行为表现到主流理论、从诊断到矫正都进行了系统的论述，真实全面地反映了我们目前对自闭症的认知。并且，她直面的是目前与自闭症最相关的问题，例如：

- 目前我们能多早诊断出自闭症？
- 为什么自闭症的表现如此复杂多样？
- 自闭症的成因是什么？和后天养育有关系吗？
- 我们能为孩子做点什么？

- 自闭症目前有什么理论解释？
- 为什么每个理论都只是部分解释了我们看到的现象？它们各自的优劣是什么？

我相信这些问题的解答和论述能让你收获颇多。在我个人看来，书中作者对自闭症的认知和神经理论进行了合理的延伸和大胆的猜想，显示了其稳重而智慧的学者风范。

我向所有人推荐这一本书。如果你是对心理学和脑科学感兴趣的普通读者，那么从自闭症切入，能帮助你学习人类认知和社交情绪的发育特征，深刻理解大脑的复杂性。从某种程度上来说，自闭症为我们理解人类的神经多样性提供了一扇窗口。如果你是自闭症患者的亲属和朋友，你可以透过这本书更好地理解自闭症的行为和后面的可能机制，也会对诊断、干预、病情发展进程有一定的预期，并对市面上各种骗术和伪科学说法（我相信你们看见了很多！）建立起一定的免疫力。如果你是自闭症的教育及科研人士，本书中列举了自闭症多样而特异的行为现象，及其现象所对应的可能的神经和认知机制；我相信这些全面的论述能让你获取专业见解，同时激发你在教学和科研上的创新性工作。

目 录

致　谢

我一度以为写作这一通识读本应该易如反掌，一鼓作气。我错了！写作过程拖沓缓慢，有时还很艰难。它使我重温往昔，回顾关于自闭症的不同思想，不得不做出一些取舍抉择。它还使我意识到关于自闭症的确凿事实少之又少。于是，我选择了至今尚在进行的研究中我认为前景看好的结果。我希望精心挑选的那些研究能历经时间的考验。

既然困难重重，知识渊博的审稿人对我来说就不可或缺了。我无比荣幸地感谢他们当中的克里斯·弗里斯、弗兰切斯卡·哈佩，以及萨拉·怀特。他们给出了无价的宝贵提议，并对我的修改提供了至关重要的建议。我写进来一些推测性的思想，他们也没给我泼冷水。

我还要感谢一直以来我最忠诚、最具建设性的评论员，亚历克斯·弗里斯和马丁·弗里斯。亚历克斯在编辑大多数章节时，细腻敏感，卓有成效。挚友海德·格里夫总能给出精彩提议。我还对克里斯、弗兰基和萨拉深表感激，他们帮我决定这本自闭症简介中应包括哪些内容，可以略过哪些。这本书属于他们。

2008年1月24日，于奥胡斯（丹麦）

第一章

自闭症谱系

是自闭症吗？

想象一下，有一位年轻母亲和她的宝宝，她爱他，他也漂亮可爱。但内心深处黛安娜偶尔忍不住会担忧她的米基能否长成一个幸福的正常孩子。比方说，她如何能判断宝宝是否有自闭症呢？新闻中经常有自闭症的报道，每一百个孩子中就有一个患自闭症，而男孩患该病的概率是女孩的五倍。一个自闭症患儿会激起人们的诸多想象，大多前景黯淡。自闭症的早期信号是什么呢？米基哭闹较多，睡眠少，很难安抚，这些跟自闭症有关系吗？黛安娜的母亲告诉她，像他这样的宝宝很多。但她还是担心：她在房间另一头叫米基时，他并不总是掉头找她。

而当黛安娜开始阅读有关自闭症的书时，她发现信息令人相当不安。她读到有的孩子整体发育可能非常迟缓，还有些孩子直到一岁好几个月之后才出现令人担忧的迹象。可能有的孩子从不讲话，另一个孩子其实又是个小天才。如同很多试图

了解自闭症的人一样，黛安娜不仅感到迷惑，而且产生了好
1 奇心。

自闭症之谜

1960年代，我还是个在伦敦的年轻学生，刚开始研究自闭症，也是同样地迷惑及好奇。不仅如此，我还被伦敦毛兹利医院里那些孩子深深吸引了，同时还感到十分困惑。正是在这家医院我接受训练想成为临床心理学家。由于对此太过着迷，我并没成为一名真正的临床心理学家，最后成了做研究的科学家。当然了，着迷远远不够。那时毛兹利医院有四位自闭症研究的前辈：儿童精神病学家迈克尔·拉特、流行病学家洛娜·温，以及心理学家尼尔·奥康纳和贝亚特·赫尔梅林。我先前读过他们的一些论文，但那时甚至都没意识到他们也在同一家医院工作。

他们的论文描述了一些设计巧妙的实验来研究知觉和记忆。他们比较了那些被断定智力发育迟缓的儿童和刚被贴上自闭症标签的儿童，发现两种群体的差异很清晰。这些差异就是不同思维的研究线索。差异不可能用智力缺陷或者动机缺乏这些一般的原因解释。他们能如此出色地完成实验并得出清晰的结论，让我深深为之折服。贝亚特·赫尔梅林和尼尔·奥康纳已经研究出那些让我深感困惑的问题的答案。例如，为什么有的看起来特别简单的任务对自闭症儿童来说几乎不可能完成？为什么这些孩子又能出色地完成一些其他人看上去非常难的任务？为什么一个能记得许多单词的孩子却不能理解单词的意思？我现在确信正是这些看似相悖的谜题对我施了某种咒语，

敦促我去找寻答案。

四十年过去了，这个咒语仍很强大。有些问题已经找到答
案——此即本书探讨的内容，但仍有更多的东西还未被发现，自 2
闭症的谜题远未被解决。

我最初就了解到，就自闭症来说，没有任何事是它第一眼看上去的样子。一个患有自闭症的孩子对你的乐曲没有回应，并不意味着他排斥你。他不做出回应的原因要深刻得多。还有，一个孩子能记住单词和图片，并不说明他就能记住人名和面孔。最让我感到震惊的发现之一是，自闭在很多方面甚至比天生盲或聋更糟糕。自闭症儿童——除少数例外——能看见，能听见，通常视听能力还很不错。然而，盲儿和聋儿能通过特别的感官接收并回应社交信号，自闭症孩子们却没有这个感官。

难以想象**没有**社交感官是什么样的，他们**无法**意识到其他人，包括后者的行为、反应以及给你及其相互之间发出的信号。就是这样，自闭症孩子完全意识不到这些东西的存在。但是，他们的确拥有可以帮他们学习这些信号的思维能力，只是学习方式不同。令人遗憾的是，他们习得的知识与我们都认为理所当然的正常“感知到”的知识不一样。正如色盲者也有能力知晓并辨别颜色，但他们对颜色的体验异于常人。自闭症患者在社交上的体验也是一样的道理。

为何自闭症患者的学习是以不同的路线进行的呢？那是因
为自闭症发生在生命的早期，很多了解世界的社交途径都受到
了阻碍。正常发育的儿童很容易走上人类进化和文化形成的通
衢大道，但自闭症儿童必须在旁支岔道找到自己的那条线路，这使 3
得他们不仅与正常儿童差异极大，而且他们个体之间差异也很大。

自闭症谱系

最初接触到自闭症儿童时，我只隐约感觉到自闭症有程度之分，可能轻微，也可能严重。当然，其实我那时见到的病例都很严重。而如今，我见到自闭症儿童时会吃惊高功能（high functioning）病例如此之多，轻度和中度自闭症病例如此之多，经典自闭症的孩子反而成了特例。但我确信那些病例还存在，和四十年前的特征也一样。但是，自闭症现在已不再是很狭窄的范围，它拓展了很多，足以囊括非常宽泛的自闭情形。现在，讨论自闭症谱系已经得到普遍接受。

谱系是什么意思？谱系实际上是指其后隐藏了一系列不同种类的“自闭症们”。所有自闭症都在出生之前已注定，所有自闭症都会影响大脑发育。然而，自闭症对于大脑发育的影响程度可能相去甚远，由此产生一系列差异巨大的表现。有的家庭有充分理由为他们的孩子感到自豪，因为孩子的与众不同很可爱，往往在某些方面还很有天赋。有的家庭因为孩子太难管教以致他们应付不来，从而使家庭被毁。当然，在这两个极端中间还有很多灰色地带，大多数病例既有令人满意和着迷的一面，又有使人恼火和充满挑战的一面。

每个人在许多方面都是独一无二的，但他们在一些根本性偏好和性格特征上是相似的。那些谱系上轻微和严重的两端，是什么把它们连接在一起的呢？在其核心，所有谱系内病例全都典型地缺乏参与普通交互性社交互动的能力，全都典型地存
4 在行为上的刻板，以及带来一系列的后果。因此无可否认的是，在千变万化的个体行为之后，存在一种共同的模式。因此，我仍

会频繁使用大家熟知的术语“自闭症”和“自闭症患者”，以提醒我们在谱系背后存在着的中心思想。

三个病例

现在我们来看三个几乎基于真实状况的病例，它们处于整个自闭症谱系的不同部位。大卫患有传统意义上的自闭症。加里患有自闭症谱系障碍，是一个发散且非典型的病例，但这种复杂的病例其实相当常见。爱德华则患有典型的阿斯伯格综合征。

大卫

大卫三岁时就被诊断出患有自闭症。那时他几乎不看人，不讲话，沉浸在自己的世界里。他弹跳球一玩就几个小时，极其擅长玩拼图。长到十岁时他身体发育得很好，但情感上仍然发育不成熟。他长得很英俊，五官精致。家庭生活不得不围绕大卫来安排，而不是让大卫适应家庭生活。他那时极其执著于自己的喜好，至今仍如此。在一个阶段他只吃酸奶，拒绝其他所有食物。妈妈在他紧迫、反复的需求下不得不经常投降屈服，这自然很容易升级为大发脾气。

大卫五岁时学会说话。他现在上一所专为自闭症孩子设立的学校，在学校很开心。他的日常安排一成不变。我们很难判断大卫有多聪明，因为有的东西他学起来既快又好，比如他完全靠自学学会读书。他现在阅读非常流利，但不理解所读的内容。他还很热爱做加法，但学其他技能就慢得出奇，比如在家里餐桌上吃饭或是穿衣服。大卫记忆力非常好，可以准确模仿听到的任何声音，唱歌很好听，音调准确。

5

大卫现在十二岁，仍不会自发和其他孩子玩。他跟不熟悉他的人交流起来有明显困难。跟熟悉他的人交流，他完全只用自己的一套方式，不会对别人的愿望和兴趣做让步，也不能接受别人的观点。这样一来大卫对整个社交世界非常淡漠，继续生活在自己的世界里。

加里

加里上小学时，一位有经验的老师观察到他与其他孩子交流异常困难，在班级里也不能完成小组作业。加里的父母把这些问题当作他个性的一部分。他看起来非常固执，喜欢连续几小时玩电脑游戏。他问题越来越严重，学校建议他去看看教育心理学家，最终十二岁时去了医院。心理学家解释他患有广泛性发育障碍，这类障碍包括自闭症、阿斯伯格综合征及其他一些罕见病症。事实上加里被诊断为患有“其他未注明的广泛性发育障碍”。这一类病症有自闭症特征，但不一定出现所有的必要特征。心理学家对加里父母讲述时还提到了阿斯伯格综合征，他父母立刻爱上了这个标签，因为这个标签更容易跟别人解释加里的问题。

心理评估表明，加里还患有注意力缺陷障碍、运动障碍，这从他开车时的笨拙表现中能明显看出。然而，他最主要的问题在于交流技巧很差和无法理解他人。加里上过好几所不同的学校，每一所学校都说他很难管教且扰乱秩序。他很痛苦地抱怨
6 在学校被欺凌。很遗憾，他的确被欺负。加里的同学们曾努力去理解他，最终还是失败了，因为他无法区分被嘲弄和被批评之间的差别。

加里如今已二十出头，住在家里。到目前为止他对母亲叫他找工作的建议置若罔闻，仍把大部分时间都花在打电脑游戏上。加里常说自己想有个女朋友。有一次他开始跟踪一个漂亮的姑娘，她去哪他就去哪，在她家门外一等就是几小时，但是一句话都不对她说。现在，加里的家人密切关注他做出不当社交行为的信号。在他母亲的坚持下，加里加入了一个为阿斯伯格综合征人士举办的社交技能小组，并参加每月的聚会，一次不落。

爱德华

爱德华在八岁时被诊断为患有阿斯伯格综合征。他显然非常聪明，尽管这样，老师还是为他伤透脑筋。老师说，她教不了他，只能由他自己教自己，但仅限于他想要学的那方面。他一丁点也不想加入普通课堂活动，直截了当拒绝按照固定课程来学习。爱德华的家人起初没认识到问题的严重程度，相反，他们以为爱德华是个极有天赋的孩子，在五岁时主要通过读字典他的词汇量就大得惊人。他很怕跟别的孩子玩，但极珍惜成人对他的关注。家人对他非常溺爱，他似乎跟他父亲有很多相同的爱好和举止，两人都有点书生气，而且都能很固执地谈论自己的兴趣爱好。爱德华大约四岁开始搜集各种鸟蛋，发明了一套复杂的系统来给鸟蛋们分类。

爱德华如今已二十岁，即将踏入顶尖大学的数学系。他之前上的私立学校，老师们富有爱心，让他按自己的兴趣来。在学校所有理科学科他都成绩拔尖，但其他学科完全无法吸引他。他大声宣称过文学就是浪费时间。除了参加过象棋俱乐部，他从未结交过一群朋友。表面上看，他缺席所有社交活动是嫌太无聊了。他跟他父亲对话就非常流畅，回复世界各地的鸟类学家时也对答如流，但跟同龄人交流有点结巴。爱德华在人群中总是很显眼，不仅因为外形高瘦，也因为他的举止和响而尖的嗓音。但是，他已开始读一些行为和体态语方面的书，希望这些书能改进他的社交技能。

爱德华在阿斯伯格综合征方面知识渊博，而且热衷于在网络论坛参与阿斯伯格综合征的讨论。他知道自己比大多数“正常发育的人”聪明太多。但是爱德华也有常常焦虑的迹象，有时还抑郁，他因此在看一个心理医生，医生会在他离开家庭去大学的转折阶段很细心地来观察他。

自闭症谱系的三个核心特征

大卫、加里和爱德华的例子表明自闭症的核心标志差异有多么巨大，至少表面上看来如此。因此，医生必须有很多临床经验才能做出诊断。每个人的表现都不一样，依据的因素多到难以列出来，但这些因素至少包括年龄、家庭背景、总体能力、教育，以及孩子的自身脾气和性格。然而，它们还是有共通之处，这就是自闭症谱系的核心特征，即主要诊断标准。你能在一些网站上找到这些核心特征。在此我们用这些例子来揭示它们的含义。

自闭症谱系障碍的第一个核心特征跟**交互性社交互动**有
8 关。仅仅孤独还不够，仅仅行为表现令人尴尬也不够，仅在社交场合很笨拙也不够。最严重的困难表现在与同伴交际方面。在小时候主要指与其他孩子而不是成人交际。成年人通常为了平息尴尬的社交场合而体谅更多。交互性交际失败的一个明显标志是与其他孩子一起时缺乏投入。

在大卫的病例中，社交失败可能第一眼会被认为是缺乏社交兴趣，或是对其他人的疏离。然而这种疏离其实是参与他人活动的无能，严重到他从来没有要求过别人教他读书，而是自学。加里无法解读他人的社交信号，也完全不知道怎样才能有女朋友，虽然他急切想有一个。爱德华可以跟欣赏他智力的人进行社交性互动，但他避免与同伴的社交互动。他努力想知道社交规则。

第二个相关的核心特征与**交流**有关。在内心深处，交流的能力取决于一个被承认正在发生的消息。一个人必须有交流的愿望，另一个人必须想要接收交流。交流不一定是说出来的话，也可以是手势或面部表情。如果没有伴随着发送和接收消息的信号，就不会有真正的交流。

大卫有着最严重的交流问题。他学语迟，语言使用极其有限，换句话说，他想要东西时他会说，但不会用来表达感情和思想。加里的困难更微妙些，他无法从人们的谈话方式来理解他们是否在开玩笑，当他试图跟别人讲话时常觉得被冷落。爱德华则非常流利，但他并不喜欢普通人的闲谈。他自从开始系统搜集关于交流的信息，自从读了关于礼节和体态语的书，读了关于阿斯 9
伯格综合征的书后，参与双向交流的能力得到极大提高。

第三个核心特征和前两个不一样：它与**重复性的活动和狭隘的兴趣**相关。这些对很多孩子的家长来说都很陌生的特征，究竟“自闭”在何处？把积木或小汽车整齐排列成小图案，这样一两次会让人觉得很可爱，但如果日复一日重复同样行为而不去探索其他玩积木或小汽车的方法，就非常令人伤心了。这正是典型自闭症中兴趣爱好的重复和执著特质的极端特征。另一

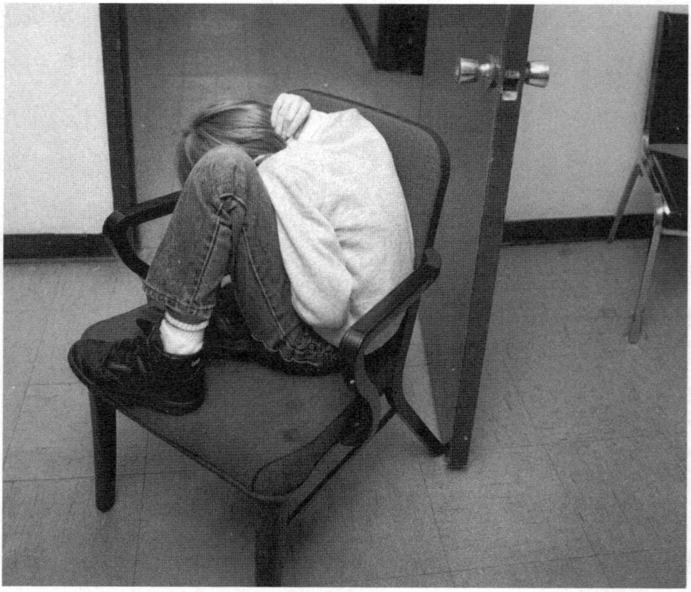

图 1a　关键特征1：在自己的世界中

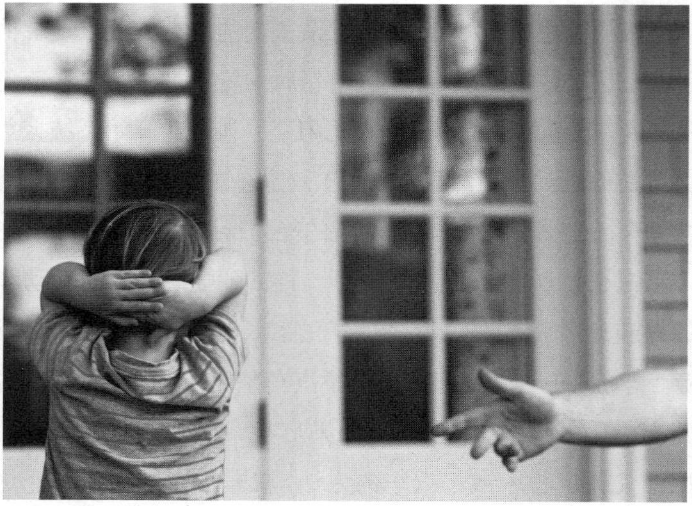

图 1b　关键特征2：不能够交流

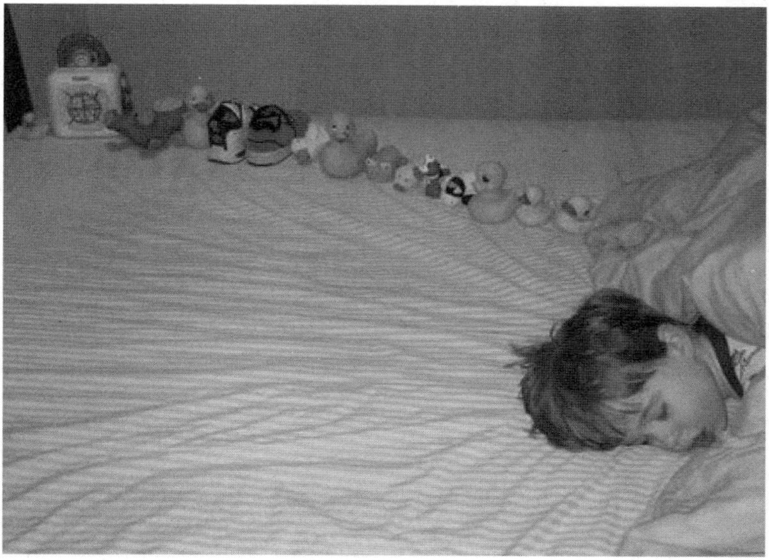

图1c　关键特征3：刻板和重复性。如这幅动人的照片所示，整齐排列玩具在年幼的自闭症儿童做游戏时常可以观察到

种看待重复性行为的方式是可以把它看作极端执拗。事实上这是在强烈抵制改变，厌恶创新。做一样的事，一模一样的事，看同样的视频，吃同样的食物，日复一日，这就是在自闭症儿童中 11 发现的过分的模式。在自闭症成人身上不太引人注意，因为在他们身上行为范畴已通过学习和经历得到了拓宽。

大卫对弹跳球的热爱就是重复性行为的一个例子，他对于印刷品和阅读的兴趣堪称沉迷。加里没有这个特征，对他的诊断因此更加曲折。他对电脑游戏的兴趣与其他年轻人并无两样。爱德华依次出现过一系列强烈追求过的兴趣。某一刻他抛弃了对词典的兴趣，转而投向数学。

前面的图片显示，临床医生究竟注重哪些方面作为幼年时期自闭症的有意义的标志或者说症状。下一章中，我们将看到有些标志性行为会如何随年龄增长而改变。

众所周知，自闭症是一种发育障碍。发育意味着改变，对自闭症来说通常意味着改善，即一种逐渐增长的能力来应对世界上令人害怕的那些事，这个世界并非与人共享，因而不可预测。重复性和沉迷性特征通常会淡化，由此对生活的冲击不那么严重。成长中儿童和他们的家庭如果能接受良好的教育和支持，这些改善都有可能出现。

自闭症何时开始？

这事说来话长，至今谜团仍未完全解开。自闭症远在出生前就已发病。在某一小点上，发生了细小的错误。这个错误发生在基因图谱中某处，而正是这些基因最终使人长大为一个具有极其复杂的中枢神经系统的人。这个错误非常细微，因而绝大部分基因图谱能顺利运作，因而婴儿诞生时看上去十分正常。
12 直到大约生命的第二年这个微小错误的后果才会显现，带来重大甚至摧毁性的后果。

为什么直到那时才出现？很可能的是，这个时间节点对建立典型人类社交行为的基础至关重要，甚至比生命中第一年已经出现的社交兴趣更为重要。这里值得我们驻足讨论一下。一个健康的新生婴儿，从生命之初开始，就会表现出强烈的社交兴趣标志。比如，婴儿们喜欢看人脸而不是图案，喜欢看真正的脸而不是凌乱画出的脸，喜欢直接目光接触而不是躲闪的眼神。婴儿们喜欢听人讲话而不是乱糟糟的声音；他们会转向大人，朝大人笑，对熟悉的大人做出异于对陌生人的回应，诸如此类。

婴儿是如此高度社交化的生命，这是有原因的。在数千年的进化过程中，婴儿们完全依赖其他人类才能生存。然而，他们早早展现出社交天赋却是单方面的。他们哭、看、笑、咿呀学语，所有这些行为都可以作为有力的社交信号传递给母亲们。比如说，哭会确保他们得到食物和安抚。但是，在生命第一年末左右，人类社交发展似乎有个里程碑式改变。这个改变与总体身心发展的里程碑改变是同步的。婴儿开始学步，开始说话。神奇的事情正在发生，原先已经飞速发育但主要可能还是单方面的互动，现在被提升至新的水平：真正的交互式互动开始了。自闭症的核心社交问题就在这里。

谁都可以看出，婴儿在生命的第一年，身高、体重急遽增长，但我们看不出其大脑如何发育。在出生时其实几乎所有神经细胞都已长成，飞速发育的是神经细胞间的联结。神经系统被数以百万计的连接体（突触）和连接纤维像接通电源一样串联起来。大脑的通信高速公路正在修建。修建过程也包括去除那些不好的以及不必要的联结。随着小婴儿蹒跚学步，大脑随之重组，随之而来的还有孩子与其他人类互动的重大变化。

既然自闭症的核心是社交障碍，人们会以为这些障碍即使在第一年也应该表现明显。值得注意的是，并非如此。通常说来自闭症要到第二年才会偏离标准，而非第一年。自闭宝宝们看起来是发育迟缓，不会在社交互动中朝着真正的联合互动做出里程碑式的重大改变。

什么是联合注意力？

注意力可以是从一个人到另一个人，也有两个人故意且同时关注某个物体产生的联合注意力。这个技能被很多人认为是真正互动式交流的基础。不论宝宝从出生开始就如何有社交性，联合注意力都要等到第一年末甚至更晚才能出现。幼儿如果缺乏联合注意力，是值得担忧的自闭症标志。同时，这个行为如果孩子们不自发表现出来，非常难以诱导产生。联合注意力由什么组成？

一个人可以唤起另一人的注意力来让双方对某个物体有共同兴趣，这种共同的兴趣本身也让人愉悦。眼睛凝视可以诱导注意力，手指指着和展示物体也可以诱导注意力。自闭症最早的信号之一就是孩子几乎不会通过眼神和手势来引起他人注意。相反，孩子似乎察觉不到他人的存在。其实自闭症孩子并非察觉不到，他们当然也是完全依赖旁人，依靠旁人来满足自己的欲望和需求。实际上，孩子表现这种依赖的方式最为可怜，比如通过沮丧地号啕大哭，比如通过拉他人的手去往他希望能获得所需要的东西的地方。这些显然很绝望的努力对父母来说非常奇怪，哪怕孩子只给一丁点暗示，家长们也会迫不及待地去帮助孩子。偏偏，这恰恰就是自闭症孩子做不到的地方。他/她不会使用对任何人来说都特别简单、明显的方式来诱导他人注意，比如不会寻找眼神接触，不会用简单手势吸引成人。

雪上加霜的是，人们很难意识到这些标志的缺失。有时，大脑非常健康的孩子社交技能发展也会迟缓。孩子的性情和社交兴趣千差万别，有些孩子学讲话要晚一些。米基就是这种情况。婴儿时期他没有表现出很多社交兴趣，有时被叫到名字时他似乎察觉不到。这很令人担忧。但在他第二个生日时，他清楚表现出联合注意力的信号。祖母来玩时他举起新的泰迪熊给她看，当她假装跟泰迪熊讲话时他乐得哈哈笑。

退化还是进步缓慢？

艾丽斯说她儿子汤姆开口讲话很早，十个月就开始会讲“汽车”“飞机”“自行车”这些词。孩子健康又快乐，十个月会走路，像任何其他学步儿一样精力无限，探索世界。他在十八个月前又学了十几个词，但自那之后他似乎更多沉浸在自己的世界里。艾丽斯渐渐意识到，汤姆自此以后再没讲过话。他甚至失去了对周围环境的兴趣，不像其他学步儿一样有任何进步。一年后汤姆被诊断为发育退化型自闭症。艾丽斯了解到，这样令人伤心的退步其实很常见，这种自闭症跟任何事、任何人都无关。起码30%的父母有此经历。 15

问题在于如何判断的确有倒退和退化？还是说仅仅在通向下一阶段发育时进步缓慢？会不会是这样呢，汤姆一开始和其他小孩一样，然后别的孩子在急速前进，因为他们进入了下一阶段的智力发展？艾丽斯认为她注意到有过一个明显的改变，而且她为可能触发汤姆改变的事情非常愤怒。她无法接受的是，一个特别健康的宝宝，已经表现过足够的社交兴趣信号，竟然突然表现得像个自闭症孩子。一定是发生了什么事情：可能是某种未知的大脑疾病，可能是某种对其他人无害的物质的中毒。几乎可以肯定，对汤姆来说并非如此。其实，自闭症几乎不可能是由外界媒介导致的。然而，只有对自闭症大脑实际发育进程进行坚实的研究，才能消除这些难以避免的担忧。

帕特里夏的例子又不一样。她总担心哪里不对劲。她女儿西尔维娅过于好动，很难带，因为哭得多睡得少。她猛烈摇晃她的拨浪鼓，美丽的大眼睛长时间凝视窗帘的图案。到她一岁后，帕特里夏已经越来越明显看出与西尔维娅同龄的孩子发育已经远超过她了。西尔维娅身体发育良好，但精神上似乎仍是个小宝宝状态。她对特定玩具的兴趣越来越强烈，注意力很难被吸引走。她似乎从不正眼看别人。她只在需要某样东西的即刻才向别人求助。她同样也不看她的玩具娃娃和泰迪熊。别的孩子过来邀请她一起玩耍时她扭身就走。其他孩子会指着书上的物体和图片迅速学会名称。这些西尔维娅都不会。

帕特里夏后来说，她曾希望西尔维娅在婴儿期难带是由于
16 肠绞痛或出牙，长大后就会好转。频繁的哭闹的确好转了，但西尔维娅睡觉仍非常困难。当西尔维娅没有显现出对其他孩子的兴趣，也没学会说话时，帕特里夏终于得到了正确的警报。

艾丽斯和帕特里夏的孩子经历迥异，但后来发现汤姆和西尔维娅的发育并没有多少不同。她们都从一个言语治疗师那里得到帮助，最终孩子们也学会了说话。他们上了一所特殊学校后，智力发育也有了翻天覆地的进步。

小米基呢？不是所有孩子都同样喜欢交际，他们也不是以同等的速度发育。米基讲话的确很迟，但他后来成为非常和善、偶尔害羞、想象力丰富，还有点冷幽默的一个孩子。米基上幼儿园后，戴安娜已经可以把她担心的自闭症放一边去了，因为她发现他跟其他孩子适应得很好，会在玩具屋玩，会把他最爱的泰迪熊拿去和朋友的泰迪熊一起野餐。她来接他时，他冲过来给她看当天画的画。

为什么戴安娜要白白担忧这么久，而帕特里夏要等上几年西尔维娅才最后确诊呢？

我们可以多早诊断出自闭症？

既然自闭症诊断是基于行为的，决定性的裁决只有事后才能做出。也许，以后可以做生物测试，在出生之前就可以做出诊断，但做这种测试看起来还遥遥无期。必须依赖行为的标准意味着不得不忍受模棱两可。而不同孩子**之间**的差异如此巨大，即使有经验的医师也会误诊，如果他们迫于压力过早做出分类 17
裁决的话。

假如孩子的社交和情绪发育似乎在恶化或者仅仅是不再进步，家长们寻求专业帮助时会发生什么？在过去，这条路通常漫长，有时还令人伤心。而如今，健康专家们关于自闭障碍的知识更丰富，也高度意识到早期干预的重要性。理想情况下，有经验的医师会就孩子们的发育细节非常详细地与父母面谈，同时测试和观察孩子。很快，便可以开始一个特殊教育项目的预案。出于这个原因，尽早做出诊断非常重要。

然而这也是个两难境地。研究者们有个问题：假如一个孩子在二十四个月时被诊断，正确诊断的可能性有多大呢？研究者们研究了两年之后这些诊断被确认的可能性有多大。结果表明大多数病例的确被确认，但还有三分之一的病例最终被认为不是自闭症。研究还表明，如果孩子大于三十个月，诊断则几乎完全正确。

很多人认为，尽管存在假警报的可能，早期诊断的目标仍然可取。有个解决方案很有意思，可以分为两个阶段进行。在第一阶段，在十八个月左右，可以在所有孩子身上进行筛查。第二阶段，在三十个月左右，给那些更高风险的孩子进行全面的诊断评估。实际上，筛查工具已经被开发出来，它主要评估三个信号：一、孩子能否表现出“联合注意力”，如用手指来指向物体；二、他/她是否能跟随成人的目光；三、他/她能否参与简单的
18 假装游戏。大部分发育正常的孩子在十八个月时已经能掌握这些。大多数自闭症孩子不能。然而，很多看起来表现出这些关键行为的孩子后来却患上了自闭障碍。这很可能是阿斯伯格综合征。

下一章我们将考虑我们现在如此看待自闭症有哪些历史原因。我们还会看一下在孩子发育成人过程中自闭症表现的
19 变化。

第二章

面目多变的自闭症

一点历史知识

一百年前，自闭症还不为人知，连名字都不存在。当然，自闭这种状况是存在的，过去几百年来的记录证据确凿。然而，详尽描述疑似病例的文献少之又少。给这种状况命名的是两个人：利奥·坎纳（1894—1981）和汉斯·阿斯伯格（1906—1980）。他们在第二次世界大战中期的1940年代初同时给出命名。那时大多数人的注意力并不在此；确实，整个世界都在混乱中。直到1950年代末和1960年代，人类才整体从战争中恢复，就在这时，一些家长和专家们开始辨认出孩子当中的自闭症。这开始于欧洲和美国，并零星地扩散到世界其他地区。然而，又过了三十年，普通大众才从媒体上听说自闭症。

自闭症的历史并没有结束。坎纳对自闭症特点的鼓舞人心的描绘产生了非凡的影响。这些孩子长相俊美，才华横溢，但他们心神不安，有严重的学习问题。这些特征令人费解，因此具

有影响力的杜撰产生了，这不足为奇。杜撰是这么说的：一些
20 孩子遭遇抛弃，创伤如此严重，只得从敌对的外部世界撤退。撤退得非常彻底，以至于无可逆转，除非进行长期的心理治疗。只是，心理治疗也不能达到理想的效果。渐渐地，一些切实可行的思想传播开来，并成功改善了这些孩子和他们家庭的生活质量。这些想法中最有益也最明显的就是特殊教育。

1964年，伯纳德·里姆兰德关于自闭症的书带来一股清新空气。它超越了当时已被科学家们在许多医学和心理学中心采用的方法。这些科学家细致地分析了自闭症孩子的认知能力，如说话和语言、觉知和记忆。他们发现孩子们有优势、有弱点，并推翻了两种思想：一、自闭症孩子有全面的精神障碍；二、他们拥有神秘的高智商。很明显，他们两方面都有一点，这个看似自相矛盾的模式似乎是自闭症的标志。1971年，《自闭症与儿童精神分裂症杂志》首次出版，现在更名为《自闭症与发育性障碍杂志》。那时自闭症还不为人知且被认为非常罕见。没有人预见到将来人们会对此兴趣浓厚，会有连篇累牍的研究报告，以至于后来又创立了几份专业杂志。

不仅研究论文数量增长，病例数量也急遽上升。所有这些都跟人们关于自闭症的意识提高，以及自闭症谱系范围拓宽有关系。1990年代后，阿斯伯格综合征的标签已经耳熟能详。阿斯伯格综合征的原型是智商极高但有社交障碍且兴趣古怪的个体。这类新原型很快就被人们和过去的疯狂天才的形象混淆起来。有种思想以不可思议的速度传播开来：我们很多人，尤其是男性，都有自闭症特征。也就是说，他们缺乏社交敏感性，有沉迷于其中的兴趣。自闭症谱系的边界仍在变动。在自闭症障碍

的各种变体和完全正常的性格差异之间，到底有没有一条清晰 21
的界限呢？这是我们现在需要解决的问题之一。

循着伟大先驱的足迹

就个人而言，我在一生中亲历了这段历史的大部分。我接受了自闭症概念的变化，也注意到确诊为自闭症的孩童和成人数量的迅猛增长。自鲜为人知和界限模糊始，自闭症已成为人们熟稔的话题。

我是通过迈克尔·拉特首次接触自闭症的。他教过我及好几代学生关于正常和异常发育的基本问题。他的思想塑造了自闭症的概念，传播了自闭症的意识。拉特对自闭症研究的贡献广泛而突出，影响深远。其中两个贡献尤为值得一提：他创立了现在全世界广泛使用的诊断评估的工具；并且，他还实施了对自闭症基因的首批研究。

洛娜·温是我的另一位导师。她有一个自闭症女儿，对自闭症有最深入的了解。我对她的经历以及她当时关于自闭症非常革命性的理念再了解不过。通过对各类残障儿童的研究，她意识到囊括了自闭症障碍整个谱系的有三个致命障碍——社交、交流和想象力的“三合一”障碍。与此同时，她还意识到，社交障碍有不同变体——疏离型、被动型和古怪型。她还是阿斯伯格综合征的第一批研究者之一。

贝亚特·赫尔梅林（1919—2006）和尼尔·奥康纳（1918—
1997）的实验性研究是我将在本书中讲述的心理学研究的基 22
础。他们的终极目标是把行为与大脑联系起来，因此他们改进了神经心理学的方法来研究儿童。他们创立了一种方法来研究认知能力，如语言、知觉和记忆方面的障碍。他们的革新之一是把实验组和另一组孩子“配对”，在一个测试中他们表现相同，然后来对比另一测试的结果。他们意识到，只有当你期望孩子们表现相似时，所发现的不同之处才有意思。比如说，他们发现，记忆一堆零碎的词语跟其他孩子一样好的自闭症孩子，记忆完整的句子要差得多。这为解开他们的思维之谜提供了重要线索。

除这些专业导师外，我一直以来也从很多自闭症孩子的父母们那里学习。最早读到的自传式叙述来自克拉拉·克莱本·帕克，我从中极受启发。在自闭症历史上，家长们才是真正的英雄。他们努力争取服务和提升研究水平，为孩子们做出了真正的贡献。我私以为的英雄是一个天赋极高的自闭症男孩的母亲——玛格丽特·杜威。我和她通信数十年。她慷慨地向我倾诉她儿子杰克生活中的困难和成功之处。她的事例、问题和批判不断地促使我澄清观念。

在1960年代和1970年代，人们的自闭症意识还很淡。正是一小群家长在美国和英国的全国协会上的出席，才大大提高了人们的意识。在伦敦，这些家长还帮助建立起第一所为自闭症孩子提供特殊教育的学校。校领导是一位天才老师，名叫西比尔·埃尔加。她仔细观察每一个孩子能学些什么，给出简单、清晰的指导，加上视觉辅助，鼓励体育锻炼。我常去这所学校，也许它最出色的地方在于宁静的环境和高度结构化而又坚定的教
23 学方式，老师们又极富爱心。

学校里的孩子们也同样是先驱者。他们表现出的细节与坎纳和阿斯伯格描述的病例极为相似。很多孩子不讲话，但会

重复周围大人们的一些单词或短语。所有孩子测出的智商都很低，但同时他们很多人表现出非凡的天赋。有个女孩唱歌嗓音甜美，有个男孩能画出令人赞叹的画作。还有个孩子不会讲话，但对质数的认识让人惊叹。所有孩子似乎都从体育活动中获益，所有孩子都参加音乐演奏。然而也很明显，这些孩子终身需要别人的帮助。

紧迫的实际问题：能为孩子们做些什么？

那时人们实际上不知道自闭症孩子们长大后将会发生什么事。现在我们知道的是，自闭症孩子会成长为自闭症成人。他们仍然需要一个强有力的结构和安宁的环境。为有自闭症和智力迟缓的孩子们（其行为往往极为让人头疼）开发出适当的教育才是当务之急。在1960年代，人们初步尝试了一些非常有争议的理念，如今已经习以为常。它们基于学习理论的科学原则，被称作行为疗法和行为修正。简而言之，想要的行为被奖励，不得当的行为被忽视和扣除奖励。如果这样的管理规则被系统采用，想要的行为会越来越多，不得当的行为会减少。这些手段成功处理了一些让人头痛的问题，如不停撞头来自残，使得他们为人们接受，甚至大受欢迎。

伊瓦尔·洛瓦斯在加利福尼亚州创立了一个运动，运动中使用的方法逐渐演变为现在为人们所知的ABA法，即应用行
为分析法（Applied Behavioural Analysis）。典型的ABA使 24
用强化一对一训练课程。但是不那么强化的做法似乎也同样成功，与那些强调和孩子们进行温暖的情感接触的做法差不多。所有这些做法都能带来令人惊奇的变化。虽然表现得微

乎其微，但行为明显得到了加强。例如，有家长跟我描述他们年幼的儿子如何逐渐在六周的课程里学会说话。起初他仅能轻轻吹气，然后吹气力度增强，能吹灭蜡烛。很快他就能发出几个耳语低音。最终他完成突破发出一个音节，以至发出一个单词。对父母来说这简直是奇迹，而这已经在很多孩子身上实现了。

还有些其他方法，目的是建立补偿和应对策略，而不是塑造和改变行为。在北卡罗莱纳州，埃里克·舍普勒（1927—2006）建造了一个中心来评估和改良有关自闭症和严重学习障碍的行为困难。他的方法强调高度结构化的时间表，用具体而又富有想象力的方式使用图片。这个方法被称为TEACCH，现已传遍世界。你能看见在几乎所有的自闭症孩子学校里，以及在为自闭症成人开办的中心里，他们都使用典型的视觉辅助，在清晰的时间表上描绘一系列的活动。孩子或成人知道他们随时可以核对自己的时间表，以知道自己在一天中的进程，也知道接下来该做什么。这有非常巨大的强化效果，还可以作为重要辅助措施来组织工作和娱乐。实际上，不同的技术是齐头并进的，它们既改变行为也适应无法改变的行为。

自闭症的多面性

一度人们以为自闭症总是跟学习障碍，或者精神障碍联系在一起，而这两种障碍总暗示大脑有病理性改变而导致低智商。近来的研究已改变了这一看法。现在自闭症谱系的情形完全包
25 括了那些即使用标准智力测试来评估也没有智力缺陷的情况。目前确诊的自闭症中，低智商大约占到50%的病例，另外50%则

拥有平均甚至极高的智力。

学习困难合并自闭症

严重的智力障碍是由于严重的大脑异常，而这几乎肯定也会限制情感和社交能力。这是大致影响。然而，大脑异常也有些特别的影响。在自闭症中可以看出这个特别影响。这里情感和社交能力完全不按常理，也远低于其他认知能力。大卫的情况就是很好的例证。然而，如果所有能力都偏低，就几乎不可能有一种能力显得特别低了。

非常神奇的是，不是所有有普遍学习障碍或者精神障碍的孩子都有社交困难。在有些病例，尤其是威廉姆斯综合征中，社交兴趣和能力还远远**优于**其他能力。你能感觉到有回应的交流。这些孩子会先进行社交接触，也试图让你参与其中。威廉姆斯综合征的个体，即使是小孩子，也会凝视他人，也会发自心底地与他人互动，而且会争取保持和引导他人的兴趣。这些通常也是唐氏综合征的孩子的特点。很明显，这些病症也有其独特的优势和缺陷，跟自闭症不同。

自闭症合并智力障碍的孩子是什么样的？他们仍然是难解之谜，而且给家长和老师们带来很多挑战。他们通常开口讲话很晚，甚至从不说话。他们看起来常常被封锁在重复性行为中，比如来回摇晃，也会被封锁在极难打破的惯例中。他们更可能患有另外的神经疾病，特别是癫痫。他们也可能长得不太好看， 26
还很可能表现出非常不讨喜的行为。家长和老师们的应对办法已用到极致。这些孩子长大后仍然极难照顾。令人难过的是，人们讨论自闭症情形时往往会忽略他们。大多数人想到的自闭症都是高功能的，而不是低功能的状况。然而这才是自闭症最棘手的那一面。急切需要研究来探寻这些个体大脑中究竟出了什么问题，以及如何去改善他们的生活状况。

之所以提出高功能自闭症这个术语，是为了把它从过去人们更熟悉的情形，即缄默孤僻的孩子当中区分出来。高功能的孩子很可能实现补偿性学习。他们的智力资源能使他们发展出替代手段来学习社交技能。他们可以仔细观察社交规则，但仍不会融入复杂的社交世界中去。只要教学方式充分考虑到他们特殊的长处和兴趣，他们就能做到在科目学习上成绩突出。然而，他们的自闭症所具有的核心特征并不一定表现得更温和。超乎寻常的智力水平使得他们能取得优异的职业成就，但很遗憾不会改善他们独立生活的能力。很多聪明的高功能人士非常艰难地应对着日常生活的简单需求。

经典自闭症

坎纳首次提出自闭症时，他所描绘的其实是现在自闭症谱系中的一小类孩子。然而他发现了每个医生都能辨认的一整套标志和症状。这些孩子显得非常疏离。如果会讲话，他们多半使用刻板习得的短语和词汇。他们不仅表现出简单的重复性运动，比如拍手、来回摇晃，还会表现出更复杂、详细的刻板行为。他们自己开发出复杂的机械程序，然后忠实地一再
27 重复。他们的特殊才能更令人惊叹，比如拥有超乎寻常的记忆力。

这类经典自闭症孩子的一个重要特点就是他是个孩子——坎纳提到这个概念时，人们对于这类人的成年生活几乎一无所

知。这样的孩子是个偶像，美丽而遥远的孩子。人们对他们的高智商印象深刻，因为普通孩子达不到这样的智力水平。但，呜呼，这只是个幻象而已。随着自闭症孩子长大，幻象逐渐褪去。

自闭症孩子长大了

儿童发育会有很多惊喜。一个孩子可能长大了就没问题了；一个发育迟缓的孩子可能会追赶上来。但更可能的情形是，有问题的孩子会成长为有问题的成人。孩提时的发育迟缓通常会成为终身的学习障碍。

首映于1989年的电影《雨人》（*Rainman*），在提高公众对自闭症的意识上产生了巨大的影响。达斯汀·霍夫曼饰演的主人公就是个自闭症人士，结合了数位真实的原型。他的很多特征是基于金·皮克，他由于异常的记忆力而出名，被称为“人工谷歌”。这是自闭症成人第一次成为关注焦点。在此之前，只有专攻儿童研究方面的专家，即儿童精神病学家、儿童心理学家、语言治疗师及特殊教育者，这些人当中的一小部分知道这个疾病并能诊断出来。主要接触成人的那些神经学家、精神病学家和心理学家们对这种状况仍然一无所知。过了一段时间，人们才惊恐地意识到，那些住在精神疾病和精神障碍机构中的很多成 28
人可能是患了自闭症。

达斯汀·霍夫曼在有条不紊为电影作准备的过程中，近距离观察自闭症成人的真实状态，模仿他们。他饰演的自闭症人士既古怪又可爱。他看起来有精神障碍，行为也是如此，但拥有令人称奇的本领。他极其天真，对由汤姆·克鲁斯饰演的狡猾弟弟的欺瞒诈骗一无所知。然而他能够读一遍便记住一本电话簿上所有的地址，也恰好能用他神奇的记忆力在拉斯维加斯赢得牌局。最让人觉得可爱的是主人公的完全不自知。他不知道自己的能力有多神奇，不会考虑他的刻板行为方式会给别人带来怎样的尴尬和困境，且毫不质疑地全盘接受别人对他的刁难。这是自闭症的全新形象，首次进入公众视线便迅速赢得同情。

雨人是一个自闭症大使。但并非所有自闭症谱系障碍人士都是可爱的拥有非凡能力的古怪形象。甚至可以说，相去甚远。很多人非常难以共同生活，很多人还有其他问题。要说明的是，只有10%的自闭症谱系障碍人士天赋极高，令人震撼。当陌生人以为他们内心都是天才时，另外那90%的家庭自然非常恼怒。然而，也必须指出，在这另外的90%的人里面，很多人也有异乎寻常的显著才能，虽然这些才能达不到令人震撼的程度。

众多的自传式描述给我们提供了在自闭症谱系情形中成长的真实景象。它们对自闭症青少年有什么描述？在很多方面，他/她甚至意识不到成为青少年意味着什么。他们并不执著地坚持要自己在同伴中看起来跟别人一样，要穿戴一样的衣服和饰品。自闭症少年们保留了其他人看来太幼稚的很多特征。然
29 而他们也有正常的性冲动。有些人会意识到那么一点他们的与众不同。他们与同伴相比特立独行。有可能他们根本不在乎自己在旁人心目中的形象，而这可能正是他们看起来更不正常的原因。现在你注意到他们步态笨拙，面无表情。当然了，这令人难过，但对他们却有所帮助，因为这对其他人来说是有问题的明
31 显标志。

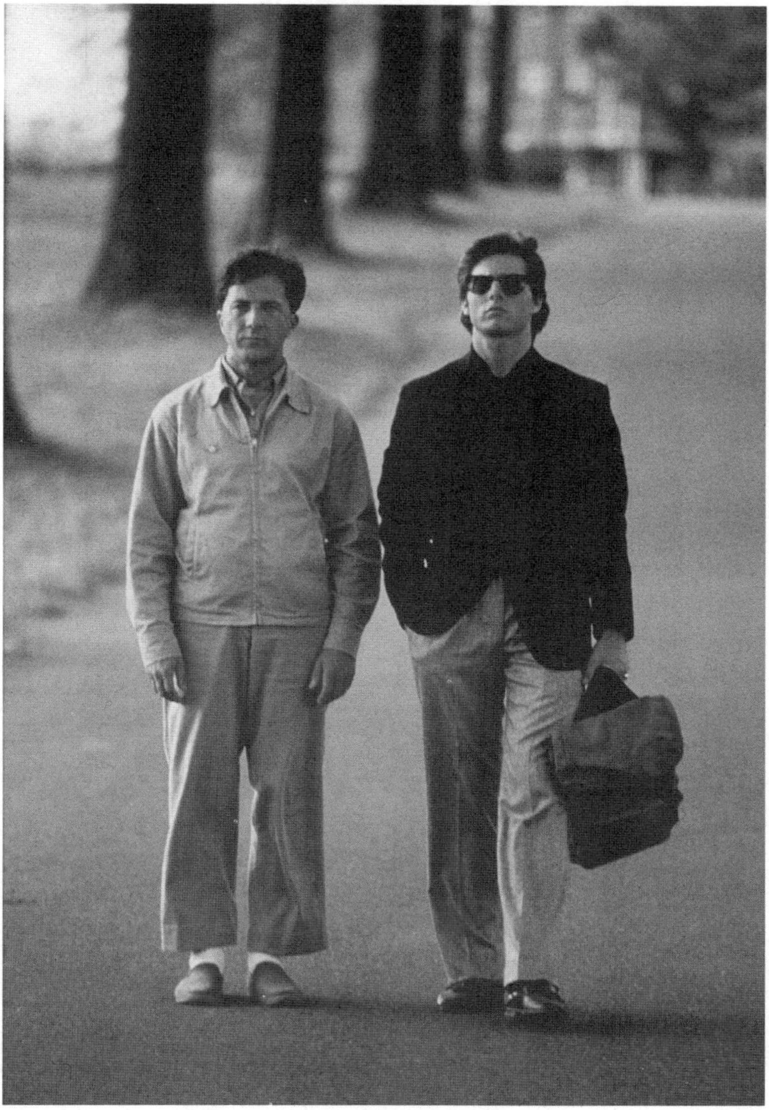

图2a　达斯汀·霍夫曼和汤姆·克鲁斯在电影《雨人》(1989) 中饰演一对兄弟。这部电影唤起人们对患有自闭症但拥有非凡天赋的成人（天才综合征）的意识

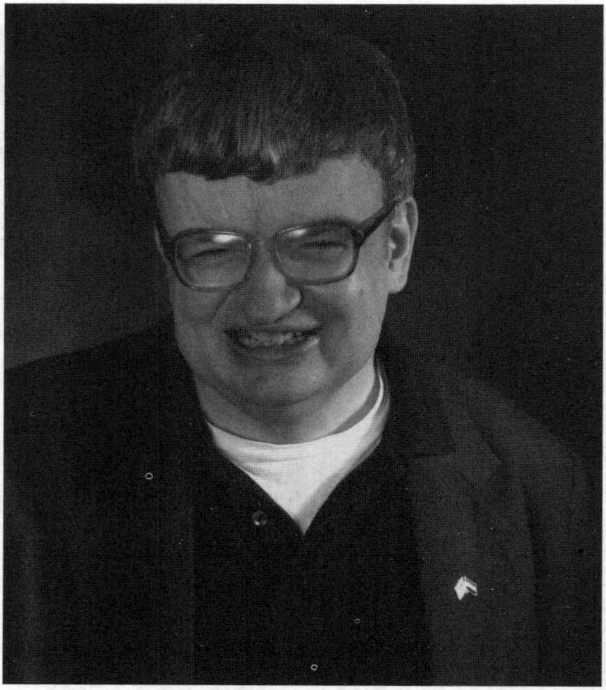

图2b　金·皮克给达斯汀·霍夫曼刻画“雨人”的形象提供了灵感。皮克能一小时读完一本书，一字不差地记住整本书。他被称为“人工谷歌”

越来越适应

第一手的资料让我们窥见令人着迷的自闭症世界。在像杰西卡·金斯利这样的专业出版公司和网络上，都能找到越来越多的资料。这些资料显示很多困难能被克服。补偿性学习有时能带来非常成功的生活，有时还包括婚姻和孩子。这一点非常鼓舞人心，因为社交洞察力的基础问题从来不会真正消失。根据这些作者的说法，他们必须一直不断地与这些问题斗争。

自闭症作者中最著名的一位是坦普尔·格兰丁，她写了很多关于自己生平的书，回顾了自己五十多年的经历。这里摘录一段她《图像思维》（*Thinking in Pictures*，温蒂奇出版社增补版，2006，同时发布于坦普尔·格兰丁的网站，很容易用谷歌搜到）里的话：

> 丰富的知识让我表现得更正常。很多人评价说我比十年前表现得更不像自闭症了……我的思维运作起来就像谷歌搜索引擎一样，只能搜索图片。我大脑里的因特网储存的图片越多，我就有越多的关于在新环境中如何表现的模板。

这段自我评价与一个有自闭症谱系障碍的人最近跟我讲的话不谋而合："现在越来越多的场合我只需要识别而不需要思考了。"

我们所知当中很大的一条鸿沟就是我们对自闭症老人的情况知之甚少。他们的寿命是否和别人都一样长？不管有没有得自闭症，身患智力缺陷的人通常寿命偏短，但原因可能各种各样。令人难过的是，原因之一是他们可能不会告知别人
他们身上原本可以治愈的健康问题。并且，他们的重复性行 32
为可能对身体有害，比如说喝过量的水。另一方面，当他们老去，他们的生活变得更重复，更刻板。很多老人会见到他们的老伴和朋友先离开，不得不习惯孤独，这本身对我们大多数人来说就难以适应。但如果你从来没有过朋友，会不会反而容易点呢？

阿斯伯格综合征

阿斯伯格综合征已为人熟知，我们应该格外关注一下。它可以被看作自闭症的一种，有相似的生物学原因，对大脑和思维的发育有类似的效果，但在行为上的表现却不那么一样。起码这是我们目前所认为的。

阿斯伯格综合征通常被认为是轻微的自闭症。但这种说法很有欺骗性。它可能是比较纯正的自闭症，只是大量学习和补偿措施掩盖了核心问题。之所以说“补偿措施”和“掩盖”，是有道理的。阿斯伯格综合征通常伴随高智商，另外，阿斯伯格综合征人士写的书讲述了他们遇到的困难，以及如何应对困难。这些困难很容易让人联想到自闭症人士遇到的困难。

阿斯伯格综合征最奇特的地方也许在于，它通常在八岁甚至更晚才能被诊断出来，有时甚至到成年才能确诊。这很奇怪，因为它是一种发育障碍。它并非突发性的，但一直存在，对这一点家人和被他们折磨的人一致赞同。

33 人们还需要进一步研究来揭示阿斯伯格综合征的早期症状。相比自闭症，它的语言发展并不滞后，相反通常还会领先。爱德华就是个例子。进一步说，经典自闭症意味着疏离感，而阿斯伯格综合征人士未必如此。阿斯伯格综合征人士往往对其他人兴趣浓厚。阿斯伯格综合征的孩子们往往把成人当作他们自言自语珍贵的聆听者，当作所有问题的答案，当作有用信息的提供者。

自闭症和阿斯伯格综合征最显著的差异在于，阿斯伯格综合征的孩子表现出极高的言语智商。这恰恰是家长们骄傲和开心的源泉，但很有可能使他们忽视孩子缺乏真正的交互性社交行为。爱德华可以再次作为一个例证。从加里的例子来看，这个标签有时也会贴在那些有轻微智力缺陷但社交障碍明显的人士身上。在这里，其实阿斯伯格综合征是指一种非典型性自闭症。

这跟汉斯·阿斯伯格有什么关系？汉斯·阿斯伯格强调过，自闭症障碍可能有不同的程度和类型，包括一些症状轻微的类型，包括那些高智商的类型。他是首批不仅在孩子身上，也在成人身上辨认并描述自闭症的人之一。他把他的病例标为“自闭精神病态者”，暗示这种情形并非疾病，而是一个人自身性格的一部分。阿斯伯格本人并没有定义我们今天所称的阿斯伯格综合征。然而，以他之名来命名这种综合征似乎是合适的。

为何阿斯伯格综合征能有今天如此牢固的地位？原因很多，最重要的一点可能是需要拓宽最初概念狭窄的经典自闭症。在1980年代，很多医生开始使用阿斯伯格综合征这个标签。伦
敦的洛娜·温用这个名词来引起人们关注一个事实，即有些患 34
有自闭症障碍的人可能言语能力非常好，甚至也有社交兴趣。哥德堡的克里斯托弗·伊尔贝里还拟定了诊断标准，以描述这类特殊的人群。这使得其他中心的医生们也能辨认出类似的病例。如今普遍用于阿斯伯格综合征的标准，跟过去被认为是冗余或非典型性自闭症的标准十分类似。它们与自闭症诊断标准几乎在每个方面都一样。非常重要的是，语言不仅没有滞后，通常还是特别的认知优势。

很多医生采用阿斯伯格综合征这个标签，表明有迫切需要单列出来。他们遇到很多符合标准的人。这些孩子和成人总体

上来说并没被严重影响，很有希望预后良好。很多父母热切希望自己的孩子被诊断为阿斯伯格综合征而不是自闭症，这并不奇怪。这个标签不可避免地受到大家欢迎。

无论是否适宜，阿斯伯格综合征像块磁铁，吸引着越来越多的病例。吸引力之一是它已成为跟天才有关的标志。所以毫不奇怪，被诊断为阿斯伯格综合征，意味着比自闭症更有意思，且困难可能更容易驾驭。然而这种看法并不正确。它的困境如同任何其他自闭症障碍一样顽固。尽管如此，阿斯伯格综合征在大众的想象当中地位特别。

从马克·哈登的书《深夜小狗神秘事件》（*The Curious Incident of the Dog in the Night-time*）[①]中可以看到对患有阿斯伯格综合征的小男孩的形象描绘。这本书已卖出200万册，被翻译为36种语言。它毫无疑问提高了人们对阿斯伯格综合征的意识。此书第二章开头简明扼要描写道："我的名字叫克里斯托弗·约翰·弗朗西斯·布恩。我知道世界上所有国家和它们的
35 首都，也记得7507以内的所有质数。"

我们直截了当了解到男孩的特殊兴趣和他非凡的记忆力。他声称跟夏洛克·福尔摩斯有血缘关系，因为福尔摩斯也极为善于分析，并且他可能也属于自闭症谱系。

故事中很多细节很可能取材自真实生活，因而提供了显著例子说明阿斯伯格综合征人士的典型特征。比如，故事叙述者克里斯[②]说，他发现自己不能理解别人，他从不说谎，他不喜欢小说是因为小说都是谎言。他不能理解礼貌用语有什么用。所以

① 此书中文版已于2011年由南海出版公司出版。——译注
② 克里斯托弗的昵称。——编注

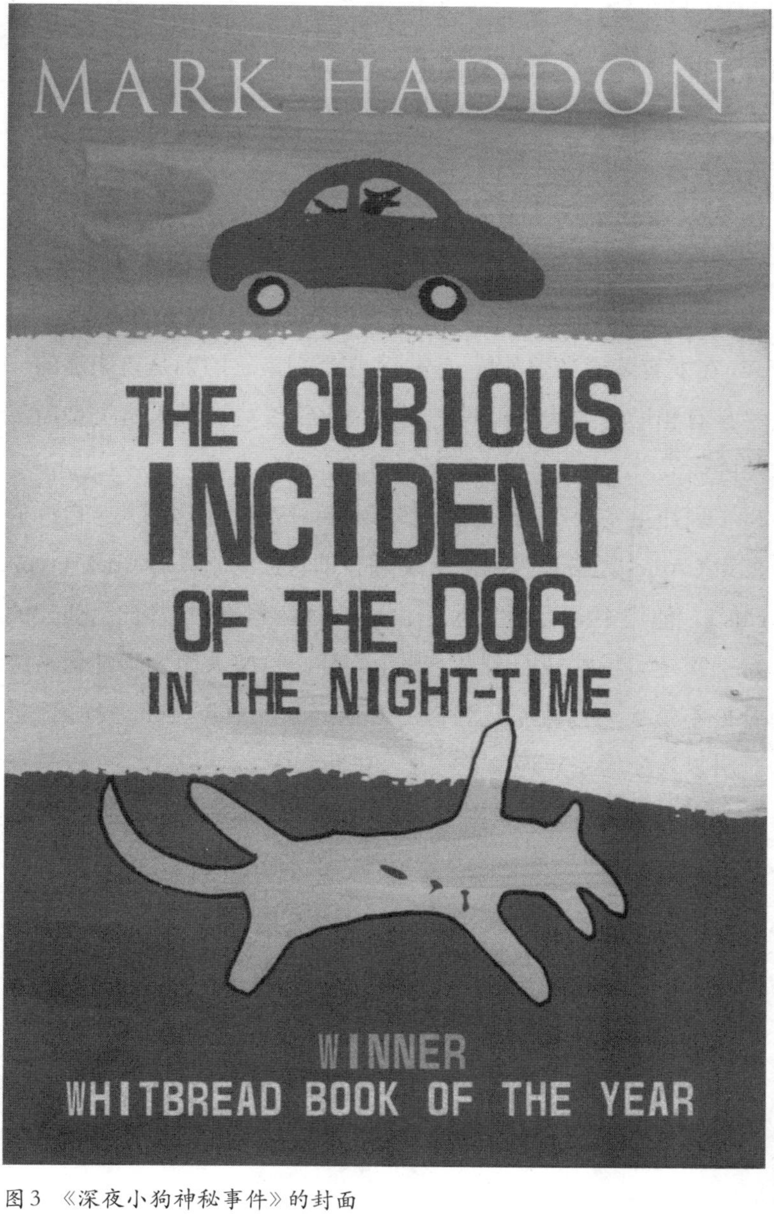

图3 《深夜小狗神秘事件》的封面

他会说“我学校里其他所有小孩都是笨蛋。我也不想称呼他们为笨蛋，即使他们其实真的太笨了。我的意思是他们有学习困难或者他们有特殊需求”。

自闭症历史的又一阶段

尽管已广为人知，阿斯伯格综合征的标签还是有问题的。我们很难预测阿斯伯格综合征最终是否能从自闭症中独立出来，在发育障碍当中独树一帜，另立类别。它的确是自闭症的一种且有相同的致病基因吗？还是说它仅仅是一种人格类型而不是障碍？

现在很多人自我诊断患有阿斯伯格综合征，这些人常自称亚皮士（Apies），自认为不同于NT们，即神经正常人士（neurotypicals）。他们不需要医生的关注，完全适应日常生活，已为他们的特别兴趣和特殊技能闯出一片小天地。这些人声称阿斯伯格综合征不是疾病也就不足为奇。对他们来说这仅仅是差异，而且是引以为豪的差异。

更有甚者，有人说对整个自闭症谱系来说，讨论大脑异常
37 是错误的，关注思维缺陷是错误的，强调行为障碍是错误的。相反，只应该谈论大脑和思维构造的差异，这些差异中的一部分代表了自闭症。这真是奇谈怪论，对那些熟悉经典自闭症和其他严重自闭症病例，并了解自闭症伴随的痛苦的人来说，这种想法
38 有悖常理。您可以坚持己见，但本书也就不适合您了。

第三章

病例的迅速增加

会有越来越多的人患上自闭症谱系障碍吗？

黛安娜担心米基宝宝时，令她恐慌的一个原因是，她觉得到处充斥着自闭症病例迅猛增加的报道。人们像对待瘟疫一般谈之色变。

可以明确的事实是，美国自闭症协会的网站表明，自1990年代以来被确诊为自闭症的病例已增长了172%。其实有记录的病例迅猛增长是不可能避免的，想想人们认识自闭症才不过七十年，自闭症为世人熟知不过二十年而已。显然，现在被诊断为自闭症的儿童和成人过去不会被认为是自闭症。与人们对自闭症意识的提升相伴的，是越来越多的病例被发现。早先很多自闭症病例可能只被列为精神障碍。

加利福尼亚州的一项研究揭示了这种变化的程度。图4中精神障碍的下降正好对应自闭症病例的上升。你甚至忍不住要说，变化仅仅是因为重新贴了标签。但其实也有其他影响因素

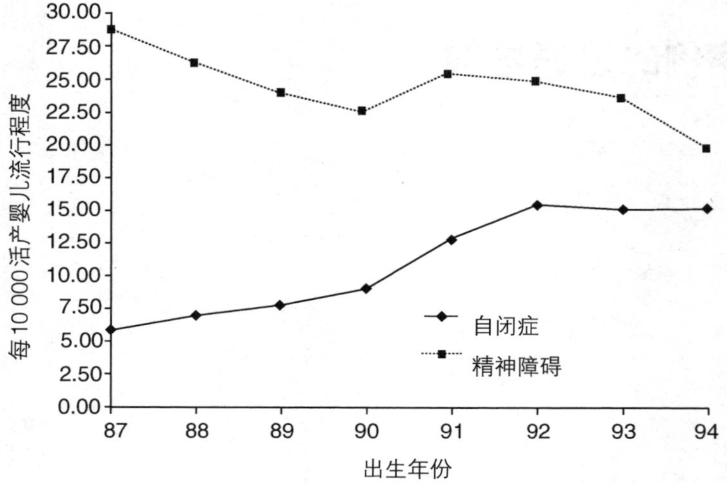

图4　加利福尼亚州诊断为自闭症的病例上升与诊断为精神障碍的病例下降

39 在起作用。

其中一个因素与诊断标准放宽有关，由此包括了很多轻微自闭症病例，以及正常智商和高智商的病例。而这些病例以前压根不会被诊断为自闭症。就算受到别人注意，也只是被视为比较古怪或特立独行。这个增长在图5中可见，同样基于加利福尼亚州的那项研究。

放宽标准

最初提出自闭症有多常见的问题时，人们只用非常狭窄的标准来辨识最经典的病例。这些标准包括社交的疏离、冗长的仪式，及对一成不变的坚持。后来发现这些标准太过严格。它们仅适用于自闭症谱系障碍孩子的一个小分支，而且只在他们发育的

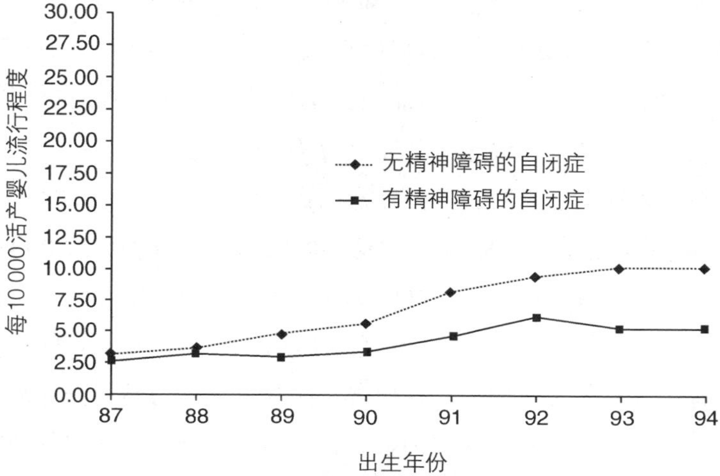

图5　在加利福尼亚州被确诊自闭症的人当中，无精神障碍的病例比有精神障碍的病例增长更快

一个特殊阶段——多数在三到五周岁间——被观察到。孤僻的孩子长大后往往会变得有社交兴趣，相反的情况也有。同样，烦 40
冗的仪式和对一成不变的坚持随时间流逝也可能增强或消退。

当在自闭障碍的进程中行为改变变得明显，当意识到个体差异的程度时，狭义的特定的标准就被抛弃了。标准放宽至现在所知的自闭症谱系。谱系包括相当典型的病例，也包括相当非典型的病例。成人和年幼的儿童都能被识别出来，智力水平各异的人也能被识别出来。另外，还有轻微的病例和严重的病例。所有这些加在一起，病例就越来越多。

现在有多少自闭症？

至今最可靠的信息来自英国的一项对57 000名年龄9到

41 10岁儿童进行的研究。在这个群体中自闭症谱系障碍的病例仅占1%多一点。如果你只看自闭症病例，大约只有0.4%，而只有0.2%的孩子符合经典自闭症的狭义标准。其他形式的自闭障碍，包括阿斯伯格综合征，占0.7%左右。

如果这个估算的1%可靠，那么在美国，一个拥有2.8亿人口的国家，会有令人震惊的200万到300万人患有某种形式的自闭症。而在英国，人口只有6 000万左右，自闭症患者也有50万以上。假定大约总人口的1%患有自闭症谱系障碍，你认识的人当中肯定会有人患自闭症。这使得自闭症是一种与精神分裂症和双相型障碍一样常见的精神障碍。但与精神分裂症和双相型障碍不一样，自闭症发生在童年早期并持续终身。

万一“真的”增长了呢——是什么原因?

以上数据令人不寒而栗。半个世纪前还没有什么人对自闭症有意识。仅有最经典形式的自闭症能被诊断出来，所有人都相信这是种很罕见的障碍。而现在，经典自闭症的病例已有那时估测的五倍之多。这是引起惊恐的原因吗？并不一定。事实正好相反，如果我们认为这种增长是由于人们意识提高了的话。即使经典病例曾经也会被漏诊。不管怎样，大多数专家那时对儿童自闭症也一无所知，那时为精神障碍者设立的机构里，也接收了相当数量的病例，现在我们知道那就是自闭症。1960年代，我在特殊医院里就亲眼见过这样的孩子。如今诊断中心遍布各地，也有更多为确诊为自闭症的孩子开办的服务机构。所有这些因素都对病例巨幅增长产生了影响。

以上就是全部原因了？我们怎么能确定呢？对自闭症状况的意识是逐步增加的。因此，我们以为病例的增长也是渐进的。42
我们还会以为到目前为止应该稳定下来了。

实际上增长的确是渐进的，最近也的确稳定下来。然而，如果因此感到自满、得意那就错了。家长们想要知道导致近年来自闭症谱系障碍病例飞速增长的**所有**原因。毕竟可能还有新的原因，比如到目前为止还未知的毒素或病毒可能从出生之前就影响大脑发育。若果真如此，找出原因就至关重要。

自闭症极不可能是由出生之后的不利环境因素导致的。我们从下一章中可以看到，远在出生之前就可以探测到自闭症大脑中神经细胞的异常。然而，这与很多家长的个人经验并不相符。别忘了这一点：很多家长描述称他们的孩子在婴儿期看起来完全正常，在孩子令人费解地发生变化之前他们没有任何理由为此担心。这种情况有时发生在孩子一到两周岁之间：他们不再说已经学会的语言，且完全丧失对其他人的兴趣。

可怕的故事

在生命的第二年发生什么不同寻常甚至可能是创伤性的事件会导致这个问题？注射疫苗！疫苗一直是引人质疑的东西。疫苗的自身特性就是攻击幼儿弱小的身体。为了预防疾病，疫苗以轻微的形式激发某种疾病。症状很短暂，几乎所有健康儿童都会很快摆脱这些症状。但也有极少见的病例会出差错，很大的差错，结果甚至会带来大脑损伤。现在如果疫苗注射累积，风险是不是会更大呢？恰好，近来引入了这样的多重疫
苗。在很多国家，有医疗政策用**一次**疫苗注射来保护大众免于 44

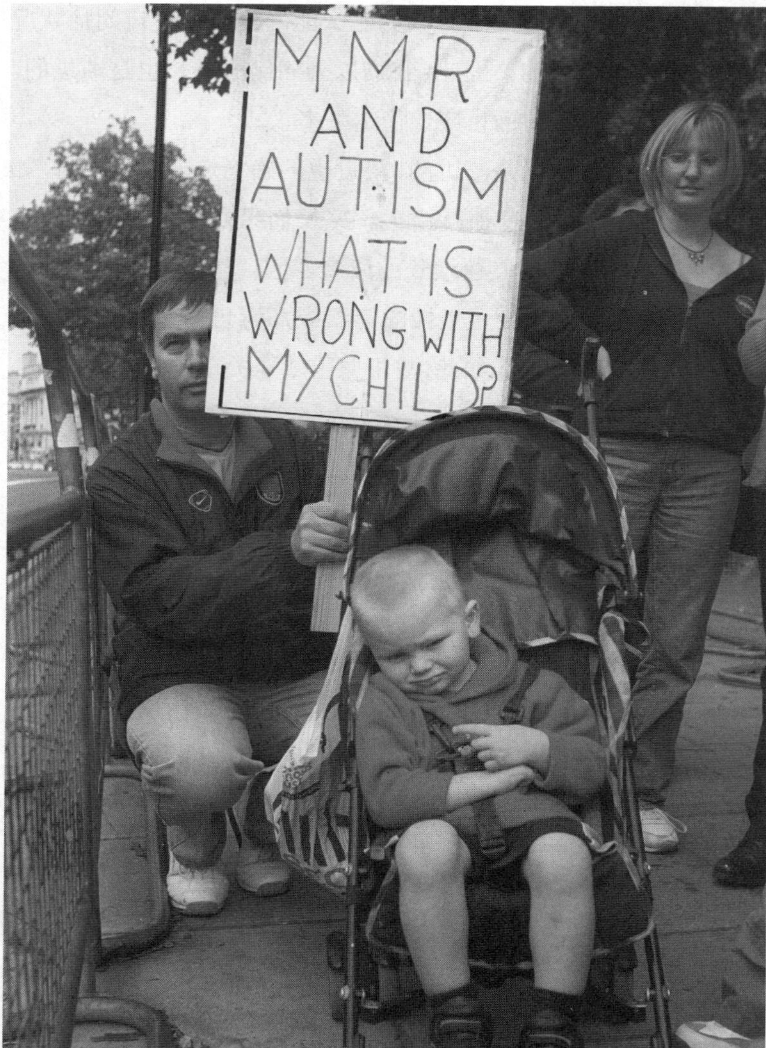

图6　家长担心自闭症和麻疹、流行性腮腺炎及风疹混合疫苗（MMR）之间有关联，图为他们的示威（图上的标语：MMR与自闭症：我的孩子怎么了？）

三种致命疾病——麻疹、流行性腮腺炎及风疹，此即MMR三联疫苗。

这种三联疫苗是否可能跟自闭症增长有关系？这个推论清晰、合理，绝对值得探讨。其实世界范围内已有相当数量的研究在大力探讨了。这些研究几乎一致得出完全否定的答案。一项又一项的研究表明，自闭症的增长远在三联疫苗引入之前就开始了。疫苗的引入并未伴随着自闭症病例的急遽增长。最后的压倒性证据是：日本在撤销MMR三联疫苗后，自闭症谱系障碍病例的增长并未停止。简而言之，这个疫苗不应为自闭症病例增长负责。

专家们钻研了个人病例的医疗记录，发现很多记录上，有人在注射疫苗之前就担心儿童发育。尽管媒体已报道出负面结果，仍然会涌现出其他疑问和反对观点。实际上，大众对疫苗的担心仍未消失。是政府和大型制药公司出来压制了真相，推卸了责任？面对强大公司的辩护，个人有没有机会得到倾听？而另一方面，律师们会不会一丝不苟地利用这个疑问去索要补偿？掩盖真相和贪婪都有过先例。既然有过公众担保出错的丑闻，政治家们模棱两可的态度就不难理解，到底站在科学家一边还是家长的压力团体一边，他们也很头疼。

但让人担忧的不只是三联疫苗。硫汞撒是汞的一种衍生物，自1930年代以来直到最近，都被用于保存疫苗和其他药物的有效的防腐剂，1999年后已经被淘汰了。汞是重金属，并且有 45
毒，因为大脑易受重金属感染，似乎这也有可能导致自闭症。这又是一个值得探究的想法。美国和日本，尤其是日本的科学家们对此非常重视，而日本由于金属污染刚发生过严重的环境灾难。通过比较在汞中暴露过的孩子和没有暴露过的孩子，研究者们能够把汞中毒排除在自闭症成因之外。并且在加州，疫苗保存不使用硫汞撒后，自闭症病例仍持续增加。然而，这种想法仍挥之不去，很多网站专注于这个事例，包括那些提供去除体内重金属残留治疗的网站，而这些去除方法本身就是有害的。

正如三联疫苗的例子一样，有些人太执著于有关硫汞撒的说法，顽固而不肯变通。他们看不到驳斥这些说法的相关科学研究。这也表明，其他未知的恐吓任何时候都可能开始，让这些抗议者们终身为之呼号。

当然，关于可能导致自闭症的环境因素，可能会有更多想法。但这些想法需要用基础研究来确认，而基础研究尚未抛出一个可信的候选因素。从另一方面来说，关于可能致病因素的那些不切实际的想法，尚未得到基础研究确认，或许会浪费非常多的时间和精力。

数量增加的更多原因

这里我们简要看一下自闭症谱系障碍的边界，这些边界现在常常模糊不清。

戴安娜所就职的实验室有个同事，儿子七岁，越来越难管
46 教。他总是做不该做的事情；他每天都发脾气；他对其他孩子很霸道，在学校几乎无法参与集体活动。莫伊拉对此无计可施，最后走进一家自闭症障碍的专业诊所。莫伊拉宣布本（Ben）有自闭症谱系障碍时，戴安娜并不感到惊奇。诊断让莫伊拉放松了不少。本不仅仅是个淘气的一直犯错的孩子。他只是控制不住自己与众不同。并且，现在他可以获取特殊教育资源，如果不

确诊他就无法获得这些资源。但换一个专家，会不会把他诊断为行为障碍中的注意力缺陷障碍？非常可能。

那些聪明但令人费解的孩子呢？与他们的高智商相比，他们的社交互动和交流能力相对落后。现在有时会迫于压力做出阿斯伯格综合征诊断，而在以前却没有人为此担心。从前这些孩子会由于能力超群而被珍惜，人们会原谅他们的社交笨拙。如今的文化当中，社交能力对成功的影响比以往任何时候都至关重要得多，因此也比以往任何时候得到更多的重视。

或许在当今，社交能力不足表现得更频繁，因为对社交能力的需求极高。可能是随着人们旅行更多、移居更多，换工作更频繁，社交生活变得更加复杂。如果是这样，更多的孩子和成人落后于社交技能的高需求也就不足为奇了。没有任何特殊问题，但有孤独和不合常理的兴趣倾向的个人会被纳入其中。很可能这些人现在也会考虑去接受诊断，尽管在一代人以前他们不会。

我们还要考虑到那些原因未知的精神障碍的儿童。在这些病例中，社交能力常与其他能力一致，都极其有限。如果仔细检查，他们糟糕的社交技能与自闭症的并不一致，但表面上 47
看可能差不多。然而，这些孩子也越来越多地被纳入自闭症谱系之下。

我之所以提及以上各个病例，是因为边界模糊会带来危险，对自闭症概念是种稀释。这很遗憾，因为研究已经成功辨识出自闭症的核心社交特征，也提供了方法来区别不同种类的社交障碍。这些很可能在思维/大脑中有不同的基础。我在讲到真正的交互式互动时，已提及了自闭症的核心障碍。

人们普遍承认，自闭症障碍标准的放宽是导致今天病例增多的原因之一。这事是好是坏？答案取决于你的观点。自闭症概念的放宽和标准的延展究竟有没有限度？当我们诊断一个人是否患有自闭症时，这个谱系究竟有没有一个明确的边界？

自闭症谱系障碍患者的亲属们呢？他们自己会不会也“在谱系里”？他们亲属当中可以看到有时很明显、有时像打了折扣的症状。亲属们身上观察到的很轻微的自闭症特征，比人们预计的随机概率要高多了。这也产生了另一种观念，即自闭症障碍的表现型范围的确更广。这意味着产生这种表现型的基因可能存在于相当多数量的人身上，尽管这些人几乎没有患自闭症的。可能这些基因倾向使得他们生出的孩子更易患自闭症谱系障碍。这种想法具有可信度，但还只是推测。

我们所有人——起码所有男人——都有点自闭吗？

戴安娜很容易发现哪些人社交和情感智力很糟糕，这些人大
48 多是男性。在丈夫身上，她发现他对浪漫电影缺乏兴趣，对足球却沉迷其中。他似乎永远在一遍又一遍刷网站，了解最新技术的小玩意和他相机的配件。这些行为是否跟自闭症谱系相关？

把你最亲近、最亲爱的人或者隔壁某人描述为“显然在自闭症谱系中”或者“有点儿自闭”，我能嗅出其中嘲讽的意味。它表达出此人的很多信息。然而对我来说，这跟真正的自闭症谱系没有任何关系。我们可能经常谈起某高学历男性，能心无旁骛地集中在某个特定目标上，从而影响到对他人的关心。他可能是个杰出的科学家或艺术家，看起来对别人如何看待自己毫不在意。有时他是个学者，并不特别有创造力，却能获得并记忆海量的信息。他总的说来不喜欢新奇，往往很古板地坚持自己的意见。

"有一点自闭"可能是一种流行的表述方式，对那些特别沉迷于自己的兴趣，不希望顾虑他人观点的人来说，也是很受欢迎的借口。它还可能是大大的赞美，隐约暗示着天才。汉斯·阿斯伯格自己也曾暗示，少许的自闭是有创造力的科学家不可或缺的一部分。他在自闭症、科学创造力和内向之间画了等号。

阿斯伯格宣称自闭人格是男性智力的一个极端变异，这样说是否正确？我曾翻译过他1944年的论文《自闭症与阿斯伯格综合征》（1991），他在论文第85页提到：

> 女孩们更擅长学习。她们对具体的、实践的、整洁的、有条不紊的工作更有天赋。另一方面，男孩们似乎有逻辑能力、抽象、精确思考、公式化和独立科研的天赋……总的说来抽象跟男性思维过程更类似；而女性思维过程更强调感情和直觉。在自闭的人身上，抽象高度发达，以至于跟具体、跟物体和人之间的关联大部分丧失了，因此适应性变化的直觉方面被大幅削弱。 49

剑桥的西蒙·巴伦-科恩进一步发展了这个想法。他提出，在人们的一贯看法中，男性智力的出色方面由拥有系统的需求驱动着。他称之为**系统化**。然而，你需要**共情**来预测他人的行为，理解他们的感情。

共情和系统化

这里可以做点有趣的事。你可以在网上做套巴伦-科恩的自闭症谱系测试量表进行测试。很容易从谷歌搜到。测试是问卷调查的形式，你只需说同意还是不同意某句陈述。例如，“我喜欢和他人一起做事而不是自己一人”；“我喜欢一遍又一遍做同样的事”。你回答的总分会得出你的全部共情及系统化分数。你已经猜对了：高共情分数是典型的女性，高系统化分数是典型的男性。进一步说，高共情分数是典型的文科类学生，高系统化分数是典型的理科类学生。有趣的是，在自闭症谱系障碍个体的亲属中，科学家的比例偏高。

阿斯伯格综合征患者在这个问卷调查中得分极高，比大多数普通人高。但千万别认为你能为自己、朋友或是亲属做诊断！我们已经看出来，诊断过程漫长而艰难，即使有经验的医生有时也会弄错。

过多的男性

其实大多数发育性障碍都是男性发生率高于女性——如读
50 写困难症、注意力缺陷障碍，以及行为障碍。为何如此，原因尚不清楚。也还不明确，是否有必要在总体现象如此的情况下去专门解释为什么自闭症中男性远多于女性。尽管如此，自闭症在能力更强的谱系一端非常极端，男女比例为8：1。而谱系的其他部分大约在2：1到4：1的范围内。综合来看，男性数量多和典型的男性偏好系统化似乎暗示了自闭症的来源。这也使得西蒙·巴伦-科恩去研究，会不会是男性荷尔蒙中的睾丸素有影响。结论尚未得出。

不管怎样——增长是真的吗？

戴安娜是否应该担心比起以前，现在有越来越多的自闭症孩子出生？其实她大可不必。没错，增长迅速，但原因也很充分。数量增多并不是谜，也不是流行病的标志。原因包括放宽的诊断标准、人们意识的提高，也包括现在对自闭症儿童的识别和服务更好。进一步说，如果现在被确诊自闭症的人不会一直以最典型的形式表现出所有症状，谁还会说不会逐渐浮现更多的隐藏病例？

但是，戴安娜仍忍不住想问，是否也有隐性的真正增长。科学目前还不能给出答案，但未来应该可以。认真、持续地监测病例是根本，警惕诊断标准的边界也很有必要。 51

第四章

作为神经发育障碍的自闭症

为什么自闭症是一种神经发育障碍？

神经发育障碍是指那些最终由基因原因导致，并在幼年时期显现的精神障碍。戴安娜想知道这究竟是什么意思。术语里的“神经”显然指大脑，这是否意味着它是生物学或者心理学问题？两者都是！看见神经发育这个术语时，戴安娜就应该想到大脑发育，因为大脑和思维从不同的角度来看都是一个东西。发育这个词让她想到我们是在应对一个动态的过程。在大脑或思维发育初期，即使是非常轻微地偏离正常路径也会带来巨大的后续影响。

随着戴安娜汲取更多自闭症知识，很多问题跳到她脑海里。如果有基因缺陷——不管涉及什么基因——你就会变得自闭吗？并非如此。这只对各种罕见的基因障碍成立，但对自闭障碍病例来说不太可能。这里的意思是，基因缺陷让你有患自闭症的**倾向**，实际情况还取决于其他因素。有些因素使得自闭症发生的可能性更大，它们是风险因素。比如，身为男性意味着有更高的自闭症风险。有些因素会削弱其可能性，比如身为女性。它们是保护性因素。 52

我们还是有必要更多地了解保护性因素。这些因素会不会让你逃脱某种基因倾向的后果？还记得睡美人的故事吗？睡美人被巫婆施了咒语，咒语让她年纪轻轻就死于有毒的纺锤，但善良的仙女给了她缓刑，让她只是睡着，并未死去。显然善良的仙女并未完全消除巫婆的咒语，但这比让坏巫婆占上风要好多了。对这个例子来说，基因倾向为异常大脑发育设定了程序，甚至在出生前就设定好了。

出生之前的大脑发育是生命的奇迹之一。所有的神经细胞都出自同一个地方，再逐步迁徙到各自的目的地。过程极其复杂，航行出问题也是极有可能的。首先，在细胞形成时会出现其他问题。最终，这些过程完成时，另一个危险会浮出水面。这就是把所有细胞联结在一起的过程。

然而，这种危险并未随着出生而停止。大脑在出生之时还远未完成发育。在整个发育过程中，大脑时不时发生大范围的重组。变化持续发生，创建极为有效的通路，以配合最常使用的技能。这些变化总是关联着建立细胞间更有效的联结。这通常被称为可塑性。

所以说，大脑一直在发生变化，如同思维一样。它随着我们的学习内容而变化，也随着成熟的过程而变化，而成熟的过程是在预设的生物过程的控制下进行的。进化已使得大部分最基本的需求得以幸存，所以我们无须学习呼吸和走路。对大脑来说，这些是自动设定的优先级，而跟思维和复杂行为有关的大脑功

能不在顶级优先之列。这里的错误多多少少会被容忍。有时发育能解决问题，没人知道原因。有时发育不能解决问题，问题变
53 得明显。难怪神经发育障碍非常复杂，非常难理解。

为什么要研究基因？

戴安娜还想知道为什么基因方面的原因这么轻而易举被接受，毕竟还存在其他可能性，比如环境污染、免疫反应、食物过敏、病毒或者细菌。在前面章节我们讨论过的研究表明，迄今为止研究过的环境原因，如硫汞撒，并不是自闭症的致病因素。其他环境原因，如一种导致大脑发烧并在随后带来脑损伤的病毒，也有过研究。的确，在某些被描述的病例中，自闭症像是由急性大脑疾病造成的一种严重后果。然而，这些都是罕见的自闭症原因，而且这种形式的自闭症症状通常极为严重，还伴随着严重智力障碍。

出于充分的原因，人们一直怀疑自闭症主要是基因编码的缺陷造成的。汉斯·阿斯伯格一再重申，他看见的那些孩子的父母当中有人有自闭症障碍的明显特征。然而，这个说法直到20世纪七八十年代才得到证明。证据来自双胞胎们。迈克尔·拉特和苏珊·弗尔斯坦成功找到了21对双胞胎，这些双胞胎每对中至少有一人被确诊自闭症。现在，他们可以观察这些双胞胎并按同卵和异卵双胞胎分类。只有同卵双胞胎有同样的遗传基因，异卵双胞胎只有大约一半的共同基因，跟普通兄弟姐妹们一样。当然，两种双胞胎的出生前环境和成长环境都基本一样。假如同卵双胞胎更可能二人均被诊断为自闭症，那说明基因而不是环境因素在起作用。科学家们的确证明了这一点。

在同卵双胞胎中90%成对出现自闭症，仅有10%的异卵双胞胎 54
双方都有自闭症谱系状况。这个发现意义非凡。其他精神障碍几乎不会有如此高度的遗传性。

现在情况变复杂了。在几乎所有的同卵双胞胎中，都是其中一个比另一个更严重，至少一对双胞胎中另外一个完全没有自闭症。这对遗传学家来说一点儿也不奇怪。记住，基因总是跟其他因素相互作用。所以在任何花园里，同一颗种子发育出来的植物也并不长成一模一样。有时，位置朝阳还是背阴、水分充足还是缺乏，都会显著影响植物的样子，影响长势，远比基因潜力的影响大。在人类发育的例子中，我们还不知道扮演种子、太阳或是水的角色的各是什么。由于这个原因，探寻自闭症基因其实就是探寻风险因素和保护性因素。我已经在睡美人故事中把这些类比为巫婆和仙女。

在某些自闭症病例中，人们已经发现特定染色体上的小序列变异。有时这些变异已经存在于父母一方当中。但这些变异仅在极少数病例中被识别出来。其他的大多数人呢？这里，最可能的是多重基因都在起作用，很难确认。

如今涉及众多家庭的大规模研究正在进行，目标是探寻倾向性基因，并找出可能同时导致自闭症结果的额外的非基因因素。然而，这些额外风险因素有哪些？看起来所有巫婆都在很早的孕期就施好了咒语。妈妈们孕期的特定病毒感染被认为也是风险因素。风疹就是个已知的例子。某种药物的未知效果也可能是风险因素。比如，酞胺哌啶酮被发现不仅会影响胎儿的
身体生长，极端情况下还会影响大脑，从而导致自闭症。 55

就戴安娜所知，她或她丈夫家族里都没有自闭症或是阿斯

伯格综合征的先例。但她仍不放心，因为自闭症的确有可能出乎意料地发生。显然，在别的家族，自闭障碍可以顺着一种极其微妙的基因图谱追溯到几代人之前。

为什么几种障碍常常同时发生？

戴安娜头脑里还有一个问题：自闭症可能非常复杂，有时看起来好几种障碍在同一个人身上叠加。这显然就是她同事儿子本的情形。加里被确诊时的症状符合好几种障碍：运动障碍、轻微学习障碍、注意力缺陷障碍、其他未分类的广泛性发育障碍，或者阿斯伯格综合征。其中哪个标签最贴切呢？自闭症谱系障碍似乎力压群症，最为贴切。部分原因在于社交和交流障碍会带来最严重的后果，部分原因在于自闭症最有可能吸引到服务。但为什么有像加里这样的病例呢？

在神经发育障碍当中符合多项障碍的病例并不少。身为一名基础科学家我已感受到临床医生们的不屑，他们知道自己同样每天都在处理多项障碍的病例。我们常用“共病”（comorbid）这个术语，意为“在病症中最重要的一种病”。很多治疗神经发育障碍儿童的专家的感受是，诊断结果其实并不重要，重要的是每个儿童的独特需求，无论这些需求是什么。这在实践中尤其合乎情理，但从科学的角度看并不能令人满意。我们需要解释为什么既有单纯的病例，又有共病病例。

有一种解释是某种初始因素的弹片效应，与干净的子弹相
56 反。干净的子弹击中后，只有一种大脑系统被影响，大脑其他部分基本是完好的。而在弹片效应下，更多系统会同时受到影响。一种可能的初始因素是大脑发育失误，可能是细胞迁移错误。

错误可能很有限，也可能更加普遍。在更普遍的病例中，它的效应可能更严重，且补偿手段更少。

然而，还有其他解释。有一种尚未证实的新思想是不稳定性。想象一下，每个正在发育的机体都伴随着一定程度的稳定或不稳定。越是稳定，这个机体就能越好地承受在发育过程中不可避免发生的危险。机体越不稳定，则它越做不到这一点。有些危险从一开始就已经隐藏在基因图谱的结构中，而另一些危险则在发育中的大脑里。理论上说，同样的危险可能对稳定的机体影响很小或几乎没有影响，而它们对不稳定机体则有显著影响。

假如我们能测量一个机体的内在稳定性，就可以检测这个理论是否可靠。这种稳定性显然是可以测量的，但它还没被应用到自闭症障碍研究中。内在稳定的机体拥有更对称的身体特征和更少的身体畸形，由此便能找到它们，这些加在一起可以给出每个人的稳定值。当发育过程中出现不利条件时，稳定的个体能适应得更好。当然，这只是在一定程度上。自闭症甚至可能袭击稳定的机体，但随后它就可能成为这个稳定机体唯一不能抵抗的袭击。结果就可能带来一个“纯”自闭症病例。对于不稳定的机体，很可能不利条件有好几种，都影响了发育，一个打击接着一个打击。结果可能就造成多项神经发育障碍。如在加里的病例中，你会发现身体的好几样物理畸形和少量对称特征，而对爱德华可以得出相反的预测。我必须补充的是，这个理 57
论仍处于推测阶段，尚无证据表明可以应用到自闭症上。

自闭症大脑

可以确定，如果某种情况对个人心智有深远影响，那必然会在大脑里留下印记。去哪儿寻找这个印记呢？确实已有许多研究发现了自闭症人士大脑的异常之处。但究竟是哪种异常？毕竟自闭症人士的脑袋里没有洞洞，没有肿瘤，没有伤疤。

大脑由数百万个神经元和联结它们的神经纤维组成。异常究竟是存在于这些神经元当中，还是在它们独自的结构和功能上？能不能用显微镜观察到？在大脑系统层面上，自闭症的印记能不能在活着的大脑中寻到？当我们在执行特定行为、进行特定的思维活动时，这样的大脑系统开始活跃。显微镜在这里发挥不了作用，但大脑系统的活动可以通过大脑扫描仪来观察到。扫描仪能捕捉到血液流向特别活跃的区域的影像。

这两种技术都被投入使用并产生了成果。在活着的大脑中，自闭症大脑在神经细胞的细微结构和大脑系统活跃水平及结构上表现异常。但解释这些异常并非易事。事实是我们还没有足够的信息，也尚未知晓如何把这两个来源的信息结合起来。

在显微镜下

极为精细地用显微镜研究脑细胞，其实是相当艰难且极少人做的一项工作。研究者们已发现，自闭症大脑的某些部分细
58 胞结构异常。例如，有一种特定类型的细胞，它拥有特别漂亮的树状结构，名叫浦肯野细胞（Purkinjecell）。这些细胞偏小，在自闭症大脑中数量偏少，特别是小脑当中更少。与此类似，在大脑其他区域，如边缘系统，细胞分布似乎更稀疏。集中分布在微柱里的额叶皮质细胞更小，彼此更为隔绝。

所有这些现象仍是未解之谜。然而，我们已经可以得出一个重要结论。人们发现的细胞自身的异常类型表明，这些异常

始于胎儿发育的早期,而非在后期发育过程中“习得”。

在扫描仪下

黛安娜自告奋勇成为大脑扫描实验的受试者。她看见了自己大脑的图片,看起来像X光照片。自闭症的大脑会不会看上去不一样?第一眼看上去自闭症个体的大脑一切正常。然而再仔细看看,就能发现诸多差异。人们发现,自闭症大脑有些区域比正常人小而另一些区域比正常人大。联结大脑不同区域的所有联结纤维所在的白质也有异常。特别是远程联结纤维在自闭症大脑中更加稀少。

扫描仪最重要的运用体现于设计精巧的实验,从中我们能看出思考、想象等过程中的活动模型。躺在扫描仪下时,黛安娜看到一系列图片。研究者向她解释,她的大脑一直处于活动状态,但相比漂亮的图片,当她看见下流的图片时,她大脑的杏仁区会产生额外的活动。甚至当这些下流图片仅仅飞快地一闪而过她甚至没意识到是什么内容时,结果也是如此。 59

至今针对自闭症人士的神经影像实验数量还不多,因为实在难以完成。一个主要问题是,在扫描仪中的人必须保持完全静止。他们不能移动头部,一毫米也不可以。还有,扫描仪很黑,噪声很大,整个过程会让人很焦虑。但是,主要的障碍还是实验的设计。不幸的是,控制良好的设计几乎没有。

例如,我们可以让爱德华和加里说说一幅照片里人物表现了什么感情,这是他们都难以完成的事情。在这个看似简单的任务里,究竟是什么原因让他们难以完成呢?如果你思考这项任务,把它分割成几部分,你就可以分离出不同的要求。比方说,这里多大程度上涉及记忆力，多大程度上涉及词语知识，以及视觉知觉？但这仅仅是一些表面皮毛。迄今为止，一些实验已经发现了任务过程中大脑活动的差异，这些任务自闭症谱系障碍的人完成得很好，但看起来完成方式不一样，即使用大脑的方式不一样。大多数实验表明，关键大脑区域的活动在自闭症大脑中有所减少。比如，让受试者看人脸图片时就会出现这种情形。

人们也能透过头骨来测量到大脑活动的隐约踪迹。用来测量大脑活动的手段有脑电图和脑磁图。脑电图测量电信号，脑磁图测量磁信号。大脑虽然一直不停发出这些信号，但只有当察觉到特定事件时才能在精确时间捕捉到信号。因此，人们可以实时追踪大脑是如何处理事件的。人们可以比较一个事件和另一个事件之间的信号，但只能用实验数百次后取平均值的方法，因为这些信号非常微弱。为了达到这个目标，研究者们会通过耳机一遍遍播放同样的音调，然后突然插入一个不同的
60 音调。意外音调出现时发生的电或磁活动的量值极其细微，它们表明了大脑对这些声音的差异的敏感程度。脑电图和脑磁图方法有巨大优势，它们可以相当容易地用在年幼或残障孩子身上。例如，人们已经发现，自闭症孩子看人脸时会有异常回应。

我们尚未知晓以上任何发现的意义，也不了解在解剖结构或生理功能方面这些实验究竟揭示了什么。一旦能把不同方法得出的信息结合起来研究大脑，我们就会知道去哪里追寻自闭症的印记。这还需要时间。

毫无疑问，自闭症大脑在不同大脑区域表现出异常功能，但人们仍不得不担心迄今为止研究结果的前后矛盾。研究者们目前偏向于这种说法：异常的根源来自大脑的联结性。大脑的最

重要特征之一，是不同区域的数目庞大的联结。大脑需要做大量工作，将来自大脑不同系统的信息整合。很可能，自闭症大脑功能的异常意味着这项工作的效率不高（图7）。

更大的大脑

直至最近，才有人提出自闭症孩子的头可能大于其他孩子的。利奥·坎纳曾经注意到这点，但他的观察一直以来被忽略了。实际上，自闭症孩子出生时的头围和其他孩子并无不同。头围差异到后来，即一岁之后才显现。然后随年龄增长，到现在为止的测量表明头围可能再次变小。这意味着什么？

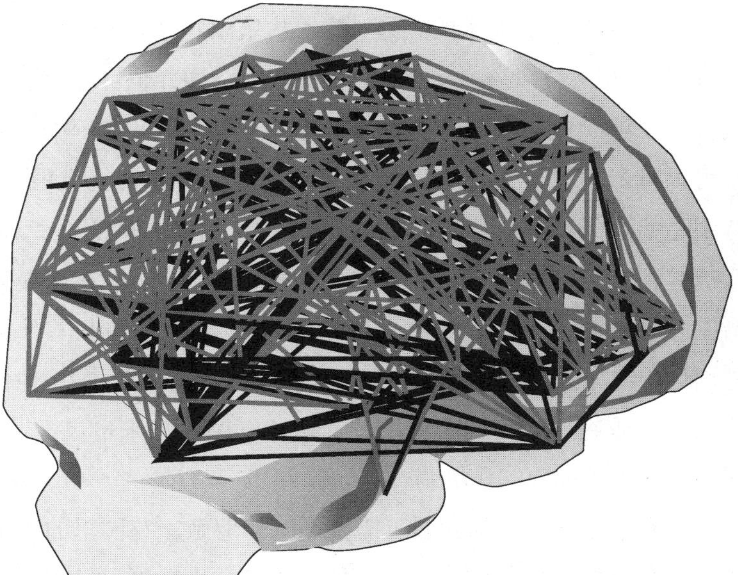

图7 大脑不同区域有大量的联结。有可能在自闭症大脑中，联结不太好。可能是联结更少，也可能是联结错误

头围，大概还有大脑容量，并不固定。人一生之中头围会变化。有研究表明，在孩提时代早期，自闭症的大脑容量增加
61 明显快于正常发育的孩子。在这个阶段，他们的差别相当明显。然而，正常发育的孩子头围也会增长，并最终追赶上自闭症孩子的头围。

从这点来说，我们仍须假以时日，追踪研究不同个体，才能完成确切的研究。但我们可以假设，年幼的大脑在发育过程中也有交替的增减。可能在自闭症中增多于减，起码在孩提时代早期是如此。大脑容量暴增的背后究竟是什么原因呢？

修剪发育中大脑的过度增长

黛安娜想到了她家的花园，灌木丛繁殖迅速，必须时常修剪，以免互相缠绕、堵住。可以理解的是，大脑同样也可能有过度
62 发育和修剪阶段。假如神经细胞数量在出生时已基本确定，那就可以推断出神经细胞的联结会被修剪。这些联结就像植物，特别是植物的根部一样，有很多枝杈（称作树突）伸展开去，以联结其他神经细胞的枝杈。在这些枝杈的接触点，存在着最为错综复杂的机制，称作突触。它们就是缩微工厂，控制着什么进，什么出。这已在神经生物学家的实验室中被研究过了，他们可以在显微镜下观察几个脑细胞。这些细胞大多来自鼠类，但它们和人类脑细胞工作机制一样。

像黛安娜一样的优秀园丁需要不时修剪她家花园里的灌木丛、篱笆和树。对大脑来说，园丁的作用部分由控制着过程的基
63 因承担，部分通过学习实现。通过学习，能把必要的联结从不必要的联结中甄别出来。我们可以想象，在自闭症大脑中，其中一

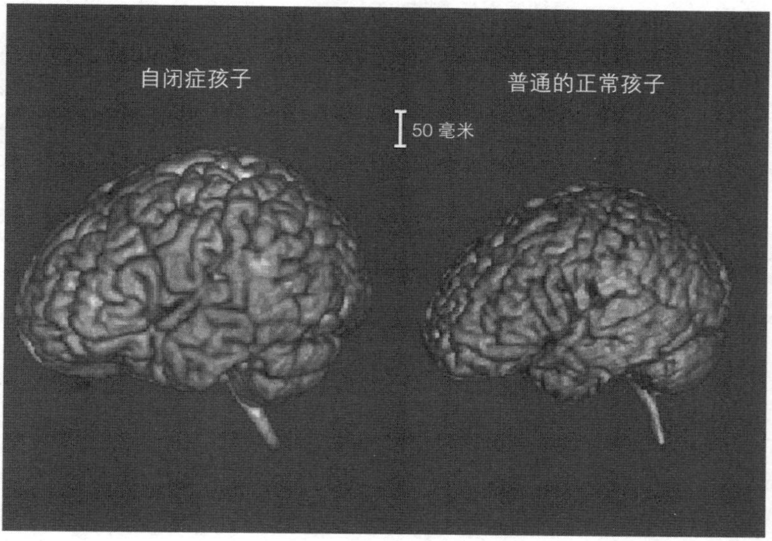

图8　一些自闭症孩子大脑袋的例子。很多自闭症孩子出生时头围小，但在一岁之后会表现出头围的过快增长。从孩提时代后期开始头围缩小的情形也有报道

个或是两个“园丁”都玩忽职守了。可能存在着过多的联结，导致了联结错误。

遗憾的是，尚没有直接证据能解释清楚究竟发生了什么。我们也还需要关于大脑正常发育的更多知识。还有很多工作要做。

一些初步结论

有个事实无处可藏，即关于自闭症成因、自闭症大脑，都还没有确凿信息可以描述。因此，本章中我着力讲了些更一般的情形，但也忍不住加入了一两个推论，如机体发育的不稳定性，以及发育中大脑的修剪。你可以读到数以百计的科学论文和书

籍研究自闭症成因所涉及的生物学因素，以及自闭症有时伴随的病症。同时，有数百项研究用结构的和功能的大脑成像技术来试图告诉你自闭症大脑的重要事实。然而，很快就会出现其他论文和书籍，它们讲述的是略有不同的故事。

从这些正在进行的研究中黛安娜能得出什么结论？首先，自闭症的成因不是一个而是很多。不同病例可能已经暗示了倾向性基因的不同组合。在显微镜下可见的大脑异常，表明了它们起源于胚胎发育非常早的时期。自闭症孩子的大脑袋是个有
64 趣的新发现，但我们还不知道这意味着什么。

第五章

社交互动：问题的核心

社交问题有哪些？为什么有问题？

我可以说自闭症真正有趣的地方并不是关于大脑，也不是关于基因吗？真正有趣的地方在于思维。我坚信即使彻底弄清自闭症的原因，我们也仍然理解不了自闭症。我们需要了解患有自闭症究竟是什么样子。

患有自闭症为何就不能完整参与社交世界？难道在听觉、视觉、触觉之外还另外有一种"社交觉"，而他们正好缺乏这种感官？生来就看不见或听不见的孩子尚能接收和回复社交信号，自闭症孩子却做不到。现在开始，我们将从心理学研究的角度来看一下通向自闭症核心的成果。在本章中，我们来看看众多科学家们已经提出的三大理论，它们意在弄清自闭症患者社交失败究竟是怎么回事。

第一大理论：心智理论

让我们回到马克·哈登的小说《深夜小狗神秘事件》。书

中主人公克里斯托弗能解决复杂的逻辑问题，但他不能理解对
65 别人来说明白无误的社交信号。他不知道谁在说谎，谁想帮助他。他为什么会有这些问题？与目前为止我们遇到的很多问题不同，这个问题是有答案的。

> ……一天，朱莉在我隔壁桌子坐下，把一管水果糖放在桌上，她问："克里斯托弗，你觉得里面是什么？"
>
> 我说："水果糖。"
>
> 她打开水果糖管子的盖子，把它倒过来，出来一支小红铅笔。她大笑道："不是水果糖，是铅笔！"
>
> 然后她把小红铅笔放回去，盖起来。
>
> 她说："如果你妈妈现在进来，我们问她水果糖管子里装了什么，你猜她怎么回答？"……
>
> 我说："铅笔。"
>
> 那是因为我小时候不明白别人也有思维。朱莉和爸爸妈妈说了，这种事对我来说总是很困难。但我现在觉得不难了。因为我决定把它当作一种猜谜，而如果某样东西是个谜题，那一定有解决的方法。

这本书只是个故事，但书中描述的实验却在大约二十年前就实施了。新理论要得到彻底验证，新思想要广为人知，是需要那么长的时间。科学突破极少发生在一夜之间，也极少由单个
66 人完成。恰恰相反，它们通常依赖很多人很多年的努力。

科学家们是如何研究像克里斯托弗这种人的呢？他们如何发现他那些奇怪问题的原因？如果读过那本书，你可能还记得

克里斯托弗只能用逻辑推理来理解他父亲或是其他任何人的所知所想。只有患有自闭症的人才不得不这样做。而我们的读者中大多数人都不需要逻辑推理，反过来我们有自动显示器。就像一个卫星导航系统告诉你在空间中位置如何，大脑有个系统可以告诉你跟其他人的关系。我们**就是知道**故事中的人或角色有愿望，有感情，有想法。而且大多数时候我们能准确知道这些想法是什么，我们大多数人似乎天生就会读心术。然而，克里斯托弗不会。

正常情况下，大脑和思维的社交部分使我们自动对他人的行为做出反应。我们不需要思考，但我们通过考虑别人所想、所需就能解释人们在做的事情。这曾被戏称为“心智化”或“心智理论”。在自闭症当中，这个心智化机制出了问题。

这一大理论做过的第一次测试在图9中得到说明。测试是这样的：萨利有个篮子，安妮有个盒子。萨利有块石头，被她放进了篮子里。然后她出去玩了。当萨利不在时，调皮的安妮把篮子里的石头放进了自己的盒子里。萨利要回来了。她想玩石头。她会去哪里找她的石头？大多数五岁及以上的孩子会极其自信地给出答案。萨利会去篮子里找她的石头，因为她认为石头在篮子里。她所认为的现在错了；我们知道石头其实在哪，但萨利不知道。

与之相反，即使是很聪明的自闭症孩子也觉得萨利-安妮测试很难。他们往往说萨利会去石头**真正**在的地方去找。他们不会考虑萨利那已经过时了的确信。他们最终会知道究竟发生了 67
什么，但要花费比正常发育的孩子长得多的时间，这种情形简单而能自动理解，但他们获知的与此不同。在自闭症当中，心智化

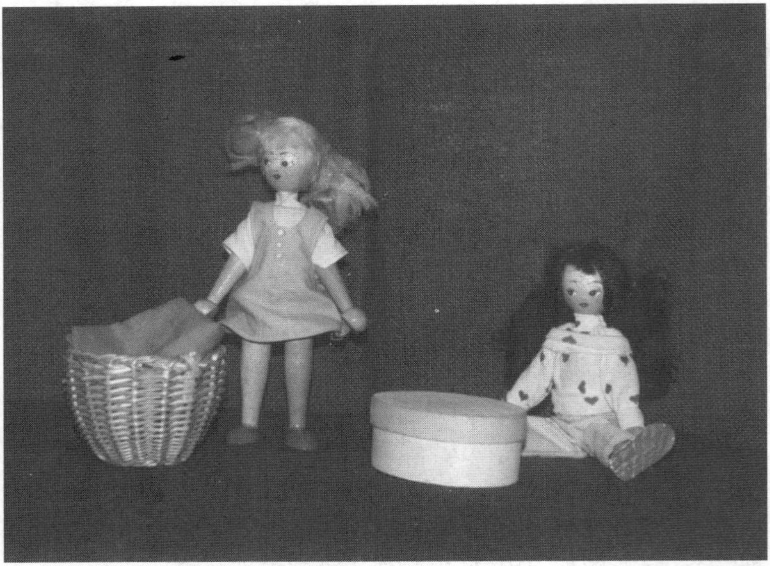

图9　萨利–安妮测试［这个测试被S. 巴伦–科恩、A. 莱斯利和U. 弗里斯(1985)使用］

从来不是轻轻松松自动发生的。一位特别聪明的自闭症人士讲过他在社交互动时的困难："我在一次互动后要坐下来努力弄明白意图、想法等等。我的确需要'离线'，事后才能弄明白，而不是实时完成。"

所以说，学习的确在进行，但通常会弄错最重要的点。例如，一个自闭症年轻人的妈妈说："我教导他当他伤害别人感情时要道歉。他也总是道歉——只是不知道什么时候会伤害感
68 情。他会一直道歉。"但也有很多病例要难理解得多。有个年轻人总是盯着别人，因为他相信只有盯着别人才能让人知道他的想法。

萨利–安妮测试是一种明显而又完全有意识的思维读取形

式，这种形式在发育过程中较晚习得。近来关于心智化的典型发育的研究，已成功找到在婴儿一到两岁之间有这项能力的证据。这个证据是从幼童观看某个场景时的眼神凝视类型得到的，这有点类似于萨利-安妮测试。比如，当萨利去石头真正在的地方而不是她以为在的地方找时，婴儿们凝视更久——还表现出惊讶。因此很显然，他们对于萨利将会去哪里找石头有强烈期待，看见结果不同时会非常好奇。正在进行的研究表明，自闭症孩子并不拥有这项看起来完全无意识的心智读取能力。进一步说，他们能否习得这项能力也让人生疑。缺乏直觉性的心智化曾被戏称为心盲。

大脑中的心智化

这一大理论已经带来从未预料到的大脑系统的发现。这个大脑系统致力于心智化。它是借助大脑扫描仪的帮助而发现的。挑战之一是制造刺激，这种刺激会引发自然而然的心智化，再将它们与不会引发自然而然心智化的刺激对比。在此对比中额外的大脑活动告诉我们，大脑的哪些区域参与了心智化。这些区域在图11中标示了出来。

结果显示，仅仅对人播放动画片就能产生这种对比。电影中的演员是两个小三角形。在有些电影中他们如图10那样互动，在另一些电影中，他们的活动是任意的。 69

第一大理论的问题

在过去的很多年里，心盲的理论得到了大量测试，但理论仍有松散之处留待日后收尾。主要批评之一是，并非自闭症谱系

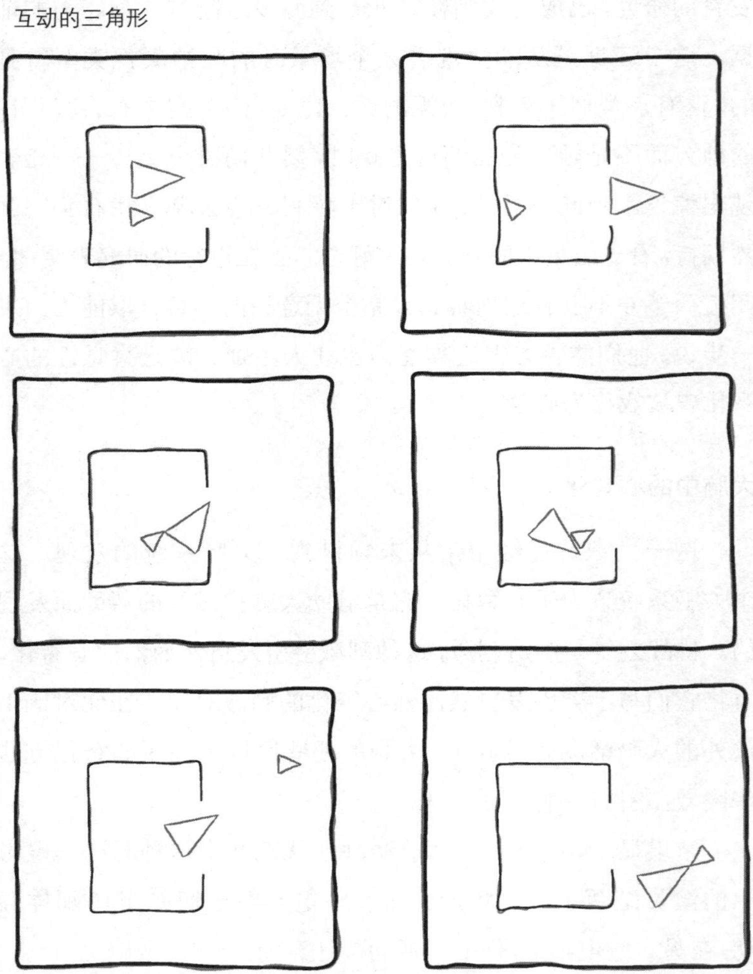

图10　运动会给人幻觉，认为两个三角形是彼此互动的生物。以上截图中的动画片段会触发以下理解：大三角形（母亲）和小三角形（孩子）在屋里。妈妈出门，温柔劝说最初不情愿的孩子也出去。最后孩子尝试出门，两人在外面开心玩耍

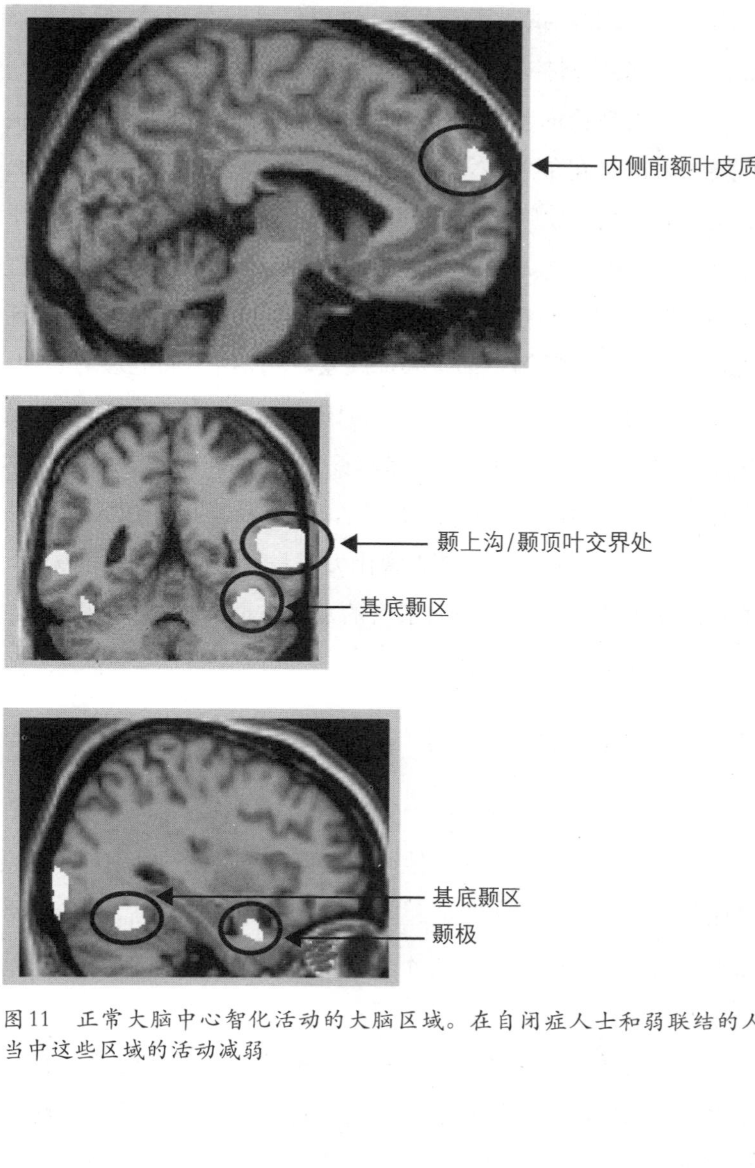

图11　正常大脑中心智化活动的大脑区域。在自闭症人士和弱联结的人当中这些区域的活动减弱

的所有人都有心智化的困难。我们不妨假定，批评不仅是基于使用萨利-安妮测试。不管怎样，这仅仅是一个测试，要想测试心智化，需要严格控制条件下的一系列测试。

这一大理论面临的第二个批评在于，那些不自闭但有其他残疾的人同样可能完成不了心智化测试。这一批评并非致命。不能完成测试的原因各不相同。毕竟，由于任务本身不同，正常发育的孩子也可能完成不了。例如，如果使用萨利-安妮测试任务，四岁以下的孩子不能完成，再大好几岁的聋儿可能也不能完成。但每一种病例中都有其他线索表明，孩子们能理解心智。另一个针对这个理论的批评是，自闭症的社交障碍出现在典型发育进程中心智化出现之前。最近对一到两岁间已经显示出本能的心智化能力的婴儿所作的研究，或许能回应这项批评。

另一个批评稍显公正：心智化失败与社交的情感方面无关，尤其是使得情感分享自动而亲密的那些方面。情感方面在第二和第三大理论中讨论得更好。

第二大理论：社交驱动

大卫从很小的时候开始似乎就从未注视过别人。他甚至避免眼神接触，有人要拥抱他时还会扭过身去。妈妈试图抱他时他的身体也不配合，被抱起时身体很僵硬。长大后他多少愿
72 意去注视熟悉的人了，但仍不会享受身体接触，而独处时他最开心。

这就是第二大理论：自闭症患者生理上缺乏社交的固有内在驱动。证据表明这种内驱力自出生起就很明显。婴儿喜欢看人脸而不是其他物体，他们要听人的话语而非其他噪声。但这

只是个开始。在一岁之前婴儿始终不断地参与进互动中，主要是和妈妈，也会和其他人。这些互动非常令人愉悦。

一个很容易观察到的例子是感情的分享，不论是微笑还是皱眉。已有实验表明，婴儿对与母亲面对面互动的时机有着精确的敏感性。在一个实验中，妈妈和宝宝能通过监视器来看到和听到对方。她们仍能愉快互动，表现出完美同步的运动和表情。如果母亲在监视器中的画面在短时间内卡住了，就会立刻导致婴儿的沮丧。健康的小婴儿简直是完完全全的社交尤物。

第二大理论的拥护者们还认为，联合注意力是极其重要的对他人感兴趣的标志。实际上，联合注意力同样被第一大理论的拥护者们称为心智化的第一个标志。可能两种看法都对。

这个过早建立起来的社交驱动，必然在大脑中有其基础。对于小婴儿的生存，这大概是不可或缺的。而大脑基础在自闭症中可能会发生错误。许多自闭症研究者研究的目标大脑区域各不相同，都被称为社交大脑。一个特别的理论是，有个大脑系统支持着我们对他人的情感回应，这个系统主要位于杏仁核内。假如这个系统发生错误，可以导致自闭症中一系列显著的社交和交流问题。这些问题的共同之处包括对他人的冷淡，甚至连 73
看别人都有困难，更进一步的后果还包括没有联合注意力和难以认出他人。

脸、身体和眼睛的世界

第二大理论使我们意识到我们都生活在一个人的世界。人，包括他们的脸、身体、眼睛和他们的过去，不仅总是在我们周围，也一直存在于我们的思想里、记忆里、梦境中及想象里。有没有可能，对自闭症人士来说并非如此？他们拥有多么不同的内心世界。当我们数年后遇到个老朋友，我们可以轻而易举回忆起当初的分别是友善的还是有纷争的。想象一下你如果做不到这一点会是什么样。你必然认为这个由人构成的世界错综复杂，变幻莫测。

以下文字节选自一位患阿斯伯格综合征的匿名人士所写的内容：

> 对我们当中大多数人都很难记住的一件事是，我们对谁说过什么，对谁没说过什么。正常人似乎能对每个他们认识的人的细枝末节都在大脑中加以归类存档，细到他们说过的小谎，都有个思维标签把它们记住。

人的世界里最重要的事情之一就是人脸，而人脸上吸引我们注意力的则是眼睛。

在一次想象中的研究里，科学家们让人们观看著名好莱坞电影《谁害怕弗吉尼亚·伍尔夫》，电影由伊丽莎白·泰勒、乔治·西格尔、桑迪·丹尼斯和理查德·伯顿主演。科学家们追踪观众们的眼神凝视。电影拍摄于1966年，当中有大量深度人际互动场景。因此，片中提供了足够多的机会让人来精确观察
74 当你看到如此极有意义的互动时你究竟在看哪儿。事实上，大多数人看的是角色的眼睛，通常从一个人的眼睛切换到另一人的眼睛。相反，患有阿斯伯格综合征的人倾向于看角色的嘴巴而不是眼睛。通常，他们会看画面中完全没有人的地方。

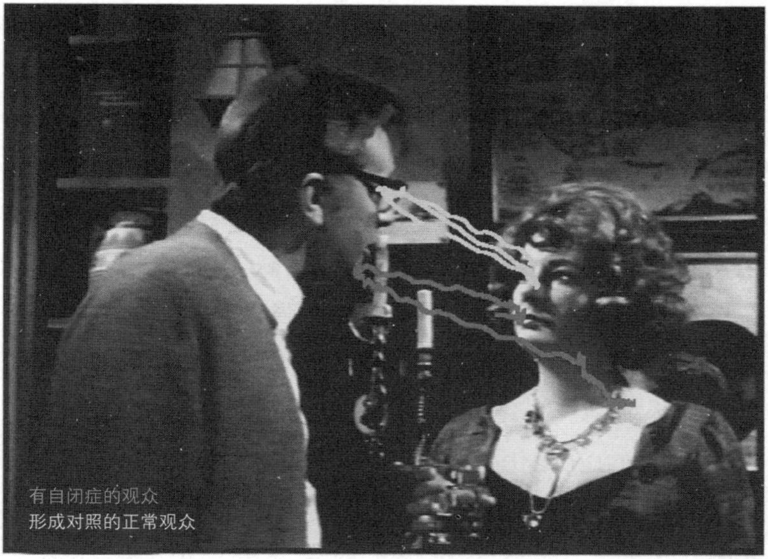

图12　电影中的场景被呈现在人的眼前，他们的眼神注视被记录下来。深色线条表明的是自闭症谱系的人的眼神凝视。浅色线条是普通人的眼神凝视。后者往往偏好看眼睛。自闭症谱系的人更可能看的是嘴巴

关于自闭症人士如何回应正在故意看某个物体的他人的眼神凝视，激动人心的工作正在进行中。正常情况下，在人看向的地方，我们预计会发现有趣的东西，尤其是那个人先看我们，显示出想要交流什么的意图。如果没有东西，我们会很失望。这个效果可以从大脑边侧的一块区域中大脑激活的增加清楚地看出来，该区域位于颞上沟周围。在自闭症大脑中则没有这种增加。大脑的这块区域在很多自闭症大脑的神经影像研究中已经 75
表现异常。这是社交大脑的关键部位，对心智化也有作用。图10展示了这块区域的位置。很有可能，与社交驱动有关的深层大脑区域和心智化的大脑区域有重合。这一点还有待未来的研

究来澄清。

第二大理论的问题

很有可能在正常发育的大脑中存在着内在机制，这些机制偏好社交刺激远多于其他刺激。有可能这些在自闭症大脑中发生了错误。然而，假如自闭症孩子缺失了社交驱动，应该在出生后不久就可能显示出来，那时强大而丰富的驱动在正常情况下已经可见了。确实，根据这一大理论，有可能将诊断自闭症提前到一岁之前。但是，如我们在第一章所看到的，这很难做到。在退化型病例中，关键标志就是丧失社交兴趣。引人注目的是，父母们强烈感觉到在婴儿早期，社交兴趣是存在的。

第三大理论：人类镜像系统

第三大理论是从帕尔马的研究者们对猴子所做的突破性工作开始的。“有样学样”（Monkey see monkey do）是一句俗语，但谁会料想这句话包含了关于大脑的一个基本真理呢？帕尔马团队的研究者们记录到大脑一处特别区域的神经元放电。令研究者们自己也感到吃惊的是，他们发现无论是猴子看见实验者的动作，比如抓一个花生，还是猴子自己抓花生，都会引起同一个细胞的活动。这些脑细胞充当了镜子。

由于猴脑和人脑非常相似，这是个极为重要的发现。即使还不能直接记录到人的大脑细胞的放电，我们可以假定在人类
76 大脑中也有个镜像系统。

观察他人做动作时，我们大脑的镜像系统会自动变得活

跃，这样我们就能准备好自己完成动作。这一点非常有用，因为它使得我们能以直接的方式来理解他人的动作。我们自己做动作时，就像我们观察他人做动作时一般，同样的神经元活跃了。

因此，镜像系统使得看和做之间建立起自动连接，这个机制使我们能理解他人动作的意义。换句话说，就镜像神经元而言，它们并不在意这个动作是我们自己完成还是他人完成的。

但不止于此。镜像系统理论不只适用于动作。想到有一个类似的机制来负责理解他人的内在意图，甚至内在情感，真是令人兴奋。毕竟，意图和情感通常都伴随着脸上和身体的动作。进一步说，大脑镜像系统出了问题，是否就造成移情的缺乏？通常，移情的定义是一种无意识地复制他人情感的方式。这个机制发生的问题能否解释自闭症的很多社交困难呢？这就是第三大理论。

这第三大理论证据还很不完善，而且对它有利或不利的发现都有。这里讲不利的发现。一种预测是，自闭症孩子会表现出不能很好理解他人的目标和由目标驱动的动作。还有，他们的动作模仿能力应该较弱。这两者在严格实验条件下似乎都站不住脚。

图13展现出一个自闭症男孩成功地精确模仿实验者的动作。实验者的目的是指向桌上一枚特定的硬币，对此，即使很小的自闭症孩子也能自动理解。他们能模仿指向的动作。与正常 77
发育的孩子类似，他们更注意的是目标而不是实验者用的那只手。他们更多使用距离目标硬币更近的那只手，不会用另一只手，即使实验者自己使用了那只手。

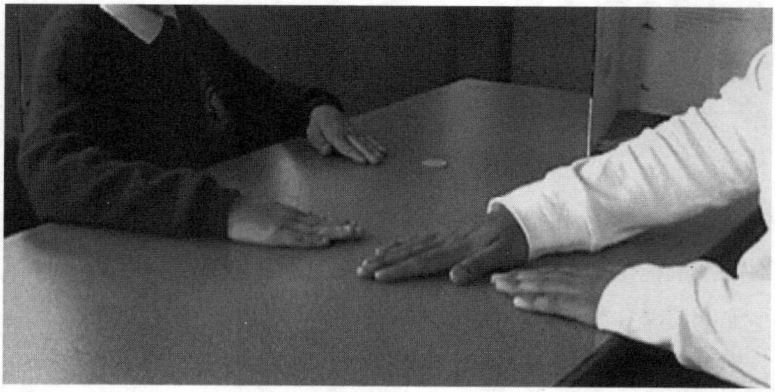

图13　手部动作模仿。实验者用任意一只手指向桌上的某枚硬币。孩子们被要求做同样的动作。有自闭症谱系障碍的孩子和正常发育的孩子表现完全一样。他们能理解实验者的目的，指向同样的硬币，但会使用他们的优势手

令人欣慰的是，我们得知自闭症孩子能理解目标，即使他们很难理解人们行为背后更复杂的动机。然而，这是一个在命令下模仿的例子，而不是典型社交情境下的自发模仿。实际上，自闭症孩子的模仿能力有缺失，他们抑制模仿的能力也有缺失。例如，这一点可以从自闭症的经典特征之一——模仿言语的倾向看出来。造成模仿异常的更深层原因可能跟心盲有关。自闭
78 症孩子很难理解在特定交流情境下邀请或禁止模仿的信号。

情感共振

我们再来看看有利的发现。在解释为什么自闭症会伴随着社交场景中拙劣的情感分享时，碎镜理论特别吸引人。当自闭症人士观察他人的面部表情和手势时，他们在镜像系统中明显表现出较低的活跃程度。这项发现还有待复制实验的

进一步研究。它会帮助我们解释自闭症中明显的情感联结的缺乏。

对社交障碍的描述中经常出现的主题之一是缺乏情感共振。我们都知道与另一人情感同步时闪耀着温暖光芒的感觉。相反，如果你与自闭症人士共同生活，最难忍受的事情之一就是他们对别人情感明显的冷漠。有一位患有阿斯伯格综合征的男性安德鲁，他妻子安杰拉在她父亲去世时极其沮丧低落。安德鲁毫不同情，并大声轻蔑地谈论岳父，说都是岳父自己的错，因为吸烟才患上癌症。他从不安慰妻子，而且对她没有完成一些日常事务感到恼火。具有讽刺意味的是，安德鲁对他人的痛苦非常有意识，但只是在抽象层面上。他一直都给非洲的一家慈善机构慷慨捐款。

显而易见，安德鲁能做到的抽象形式的移情，与用体态语表达出、如传染般让人感受到的对他人感情的移情形式大相径庭。镜像系统似乎能为这种传染提供机制。

人们所知的一个非常有传染性的面部动作是打哈欠。它连一种情感都算不上，只是一种不需要学习的原始反射。日本研究者们把静止的打哈欠面庞的图片给自闭症儿童看，并记录下他们打哈欠的倾向。结论显示在图14中。自闭症孩子受到的 79
传染比正常发育的孩子少得多。这项发现还需要在成人身上复制。现在也有关于情感的类似实验正在展开。

第三大理论的问题

碎镜理论还很新。它还需要加以改进，才能解释自闭症中哪些社交互动出了问题。和另外两大理论一样，它不能解释自

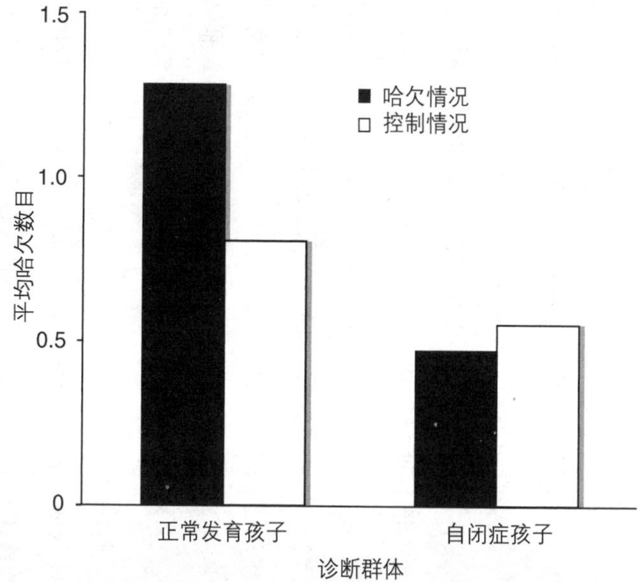

图14

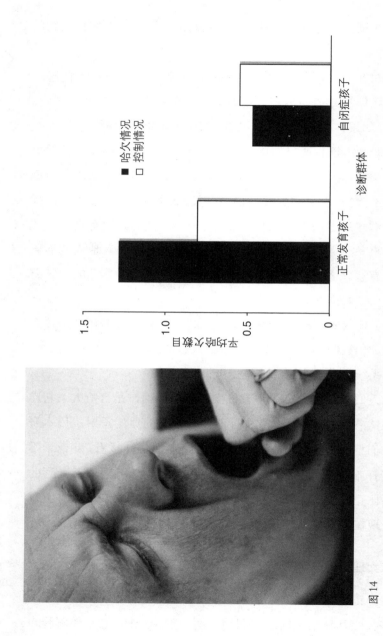

左：看见有人打哈欠，我们通常感觉自己也想打哈欠

右：与正常发育的孩子相比，有自闭症谱系障碍的孩子看脸部打哈欠和仅仅张开嘴巴的图片打的传染性哈欠更少

闭症涵盖的贫乏社交生活当中的所有问题。然而，它给出了一个激动人心的可能性：它能帮我们理解为什么在自闭症中奇怪地缺乏情感回应。有可能这个理论在未来会定义一种认知的表现型，最终找到配对的基因型。可以想象一个人展现出所有三种认知的表现型、心智化失败、缺乏社交驱动以及镜像系统失败。也可以想象在自闭症谱系上不同部位的人，他们仅切合其中一种。

语言与交流

这在自闭症中是不是一个单独的问题？还是说它是社交障碍的重要部分？若果真如此，三大理论中哪种处理得最好？

想象一下我们如何与一台取款机交流，然后想象一下我们如何与另一个人交流。一个患自闭症的人不会看出两者有多大差异。这可能是由于缺乏社交驱动，即第二大理论。

第一大理论是刺向问题的另一把匕首。交流是真正的交互式互动，这就是心盲理论试图解释的。交互式互动不仅仅是提出和回答问题。我们还总是探寻交流对象已经理解了多少对话，他或她被我们说服了多少。我们面对一台机器时则不会这么做。 81

心盲给普通的双向交流带来灾难性后果。例如，自闭症人士不能理解闲谈和玩笑的意义。我们大多热爱这么做，因为它使我们除了交流信息外还能做很多事。我们选择用词的方式显示了我们对待世界的态度。并且，我们也了解到他人对待我们的态度。他们不会直接告诉我们，但我们大脑中类似导航的装置让我们能感受到。相反，自闭症人士仅能适应信息交流本身。

所以你不要嘲弄他们，不要开玩笑，不要使用反讽。他们首先的倾向会是把所有论述按字面意思当真。需要指出，对正常发育的孩子，不需要告诉他们别太刻板地理解字面意思。他们完全能够自己理解。

交谈和交流容易混为一谈。大卫不讲话时，他父母急切盼望他能说话。他们非常确信当他开始使用词语的时候，交流之门将最终对他敞开。令人遗憾的是，这并没有发生。大卫现在会讲话，但他仍然不交流。交流之门并不需要等到解锁语言才能打开。如果交流被封锁，语言不会是钥匙。只有在意识到自己思维里有不同于他人思维的有趣的东西时，你才会有交流的愿望。这与第一大理论——心盲——切合。但其他两种理论也能解释交流的缺失。第二大理论表明，由于缺乏社交驱动，交流永远无法顺利展开。第三大理论解释称，这是由于缺乏他人情感、意图甚至动作的镜像。确实，我们不仅仅是通过互相交谈来交流，还通过运动方式、面部表情、手势，事实上是我们的整个身体来交流。身体语言经常泄露我们的所感所想，尽管我们竭力用语言来隐藏。

因此，三大理论都有能解释交流问题的部分。这些交流问
82 题正是自闭症的核心所在。

没有一概而论的社交失败

在本章中，对于自闭症中残忍且往往具有摧毁性的社交和交流失败，我们考察了三种不同的解释。但假如你认为自闭症人士完全没有社交能力，那就错了。在热情寻找这些问题的原因时，我们不能忘记他们残存的社交能力。

罗纳德曾加入一个竹节虫迷俱乐部。成员们比较关于竹节虫的笔记和图片：在英国就有1 560多种。每个路灯都有自己的一群竹节虫。罗纳德希望在俱乐部里找到个女朋友。事实上成员里真有个女孩，但并不是他想要的，因为她不是金发碧眼，不算很漂亮。大多数自闭症男士判断女性魅力的能力丝毫不差。

四岁的塞巴斯蒂安几乎完全沉浸在自己的世界里。然而有一天，妈妈注意到，他拿了个毯子盖在沙发上小憩的妈妈身上。超越自闭症谱系障碍人士身上典型的强烈自我中心主义、表达爱心的事例虽然很少，但不是没有。与此类似，共情的例子也存在，尽管缺乏共情通常被认为是自闭症的典型特征。其实缺乏共情在另一种障碍——精神变态——的人身上也很常见。精神变态是一种情绪障碍，会影响道德判断。然而，不同于自闭症人士，精神变态者善于读取他人思维，清楚知道怎样去蒙蔽和欺诈别人。

西尔维娅对别人很健忘，至少看起来如此。她没什么社交兴趣。她也缺乏心智化能力。她几乎不会去注意人，所以也很难说她究竟能否意识到显露情感的表情，能否记住别人的面庞。 83

她去参加一项研究性别和种族成见知识的实验时，人们大跌眼镜。这些成见她知道很多！实际上，西尔维娅并不是唯一一个以这种知识让大家大吃一惊的人。被测试的其他自闭症孩子也显示出与正常发育孩子同样的社交成见。例如，实验者就一个男孩和一个女孩的图片提出以下问题："这是杰克，这是曼迪。两个孩子中有一人有四个布娃娃。谁有四个布娃娃？"西尔维娅准确无误地指向女孩。

除了性别成见（玩布娃娃、做饭、照顾他人，等等），种族成见也同样被研究。性别成见还可能让人相信是从观察中学习到的，种族成见则不太可能基于亲身经历。大错特错！黑人是如何跟撒谎、肮脏、不友好联系起来的，而白人就是诚实、干净、友好的？当实验者问“哪个人偷了钱包？”时，西尔维娅指向一个棕色皮肤的人。当实验者问“哪个人有很多朋友？”时，和任何其他自闭症或者非自闭症孩子一样，她指向粉色皮肤的人。她是如何获得这些成见的？或许是她吸收了隐含的文化态度。这意味着这些态度对她并非不能渗透，这也提出了一种可能，即一些还未被预料到的社交学习类型对自闭症孩子来说是可能的，虽然尚无研究。

这几个例子表明，我们的社交世界并未完全对自闭症个体关闭。我们的社交世界究竟向自闭症人士敞开了哪一面？今后
84 的研究或许会带来更多令人吃惊的答案。

第六章

不同角度看世界

天才之谜

关于自闭症最令人叹绝的事实，也是所有对自闭症的虚构描述都会称颂的事实，就是天才型（savant）人才。这些才能即使在不说话、有严重智力障碍的人身上也闪耀着光芒。这个词来自idiots savants，字面意思为“愚蠢的天才”，提醒我们原本这些天赋是在极低的智力水平以及或许极不正常的大脑里观察到的。后来savant这个词被用来指不论智力水平如何、拥有不一般的非凡天赋的人。天赋是自发获得的，而且通常是意外发现。金·皮克能仅仅通过阅读记住整本书。没人教过他这一点。我认识一个男孩，能在一整页越来越大的数字中极快地找出其中的质数。其他令人惊叹的例子包括音乐和艺术作品。

图15给出的是一个当之无愧的著名天才艺术家的例子。斯蒂芬·威尔特希尔绘制罗马城市风光的过程被拍摄下来，他是从直升机上俯视罗马的。读者们可以从网上找到这段录像。斯蒂

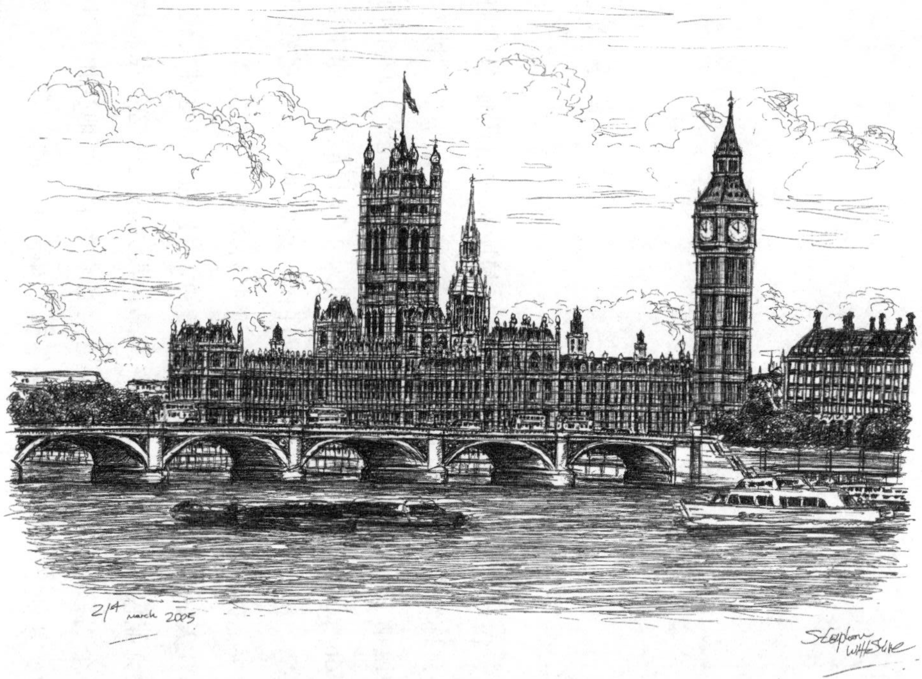

图15 斯蒂芬·威尔特希尔完全靠记忆创作出这幅伦敦市景。斯蒂芬的画作高度精确,但也很有创意,高度原创

芬记得在这段45分钟的飞行中看到的一切东西，花了三天时间
才画出完整的全景。他首先画的不是宏大的地图轮廓和主要特 85
征，而是直接从圣彼得大教堂的细节开始，教堂位于他画作的中
间位置。然后他填满右面的空间，然后是左面的空间，所有细节
一丝不苟。用这种方式他画出了非常精确的画作，就像完全忠
实地储存于记忆中。这种非同凡响的现象该如何解释？

出人意料的长处

并非每一个自闭症孩子都有杰出的天分。然而，他们大多有些出乎意料的能力。我最近在自闭症谱系障碍人士的网站上找到一位46岁女士发的帖子："我从来不知道拼图游戏应该根据图像而不是形状拼起来。"这与我研究自闭症孩子早期提出的一个说法不谋而合：有些孩子能把拼图倒过来拼，完全不借助图片的帮助。这使得我做了早期的一个实验。我邀请孩子们完成一个拼图，图片的颜色很简单。有时碎片是直的，有时它们有锯齿。我测试的自闭症孩子们非常乐意完成有锯齿边小块的拼图，对图片毫不在意。非自闭症孩子们对组成图片兴趣更大，当他们看到直边的碎片而不需要摆弄那些棘手的锯齿边时很开心。

据我所知，这个简单实验的结果与其他实验结果是一致的。这些实验中，自闭症孩子被要求听词语，词语或者以无意义的方式随机组合，或者呈现为一句合适的话，让他们立刻回忆出来。大多数孩子对句子形式的词语记忆更好，即使有点长也能记得不错。自闭症孩子并非如此。相反，他们当中有人能奇迹般记住很长的顺序打乱的词语串。

然而，另一些实验表明，自闭症孩子们极为擅长找到镶嵌在

大幅有意义图片上的隐藏形状。他们当中有些喜爱《威力在哪
87 里》这种书，比自己的兄弟姐妹找得更快更好。已有很多研究结果表明，自闭症孩子对某些任务完成得极好，另一些任务则完成得很差。在这里也许能发现他们奇怪智力的线索，他们的智力可以同时表现得非常高和非常低。

有一种观点认为，自闭症孩子关注句子或图片里可能无意义的线索，但不会关注整个句子或整幅图片的意义。若果真如此，这就是完全不同的信息处理方式。这种处理风格会不会同时导致另一种不同的智力？它能解释特殊天才的事？这些问题催生了弱中央统合功能理论，即第四大理论。这个理论试图解释的东西一方面在图16中得到例证，另一方面也从马克·哈登书上（第7页）的一个例子中看出。在这里，克里斯托弗显然没有像他应该的那样，在警察出现时非常吃惊或害怕，特别是在警察想把他带到警察局去时。相反，他注意到警察们外表的一些细枝末节。

> 然后警察来了。我喜欢警察。他们穿制服，有号牌，你能知道他们想做什么。有一个女警察和一个男警察。女警察裤子的左脚踝处有个小洞，小洞中间有红色擦痕。男警察鞋底粘上了一大片橙色的树叶，从鞋底一边戳了出来。

兴趣狭窄与行为刻板

不同的自闭症人士都曾写过他们对细节的热爱及专注细节的能力。对细节的专注兴趣在别人看起来很狭窄，而狭窄的兴
88 趣是自闭症谱系障碍，特别是阿斯伯格综合征诊断的核心特征。

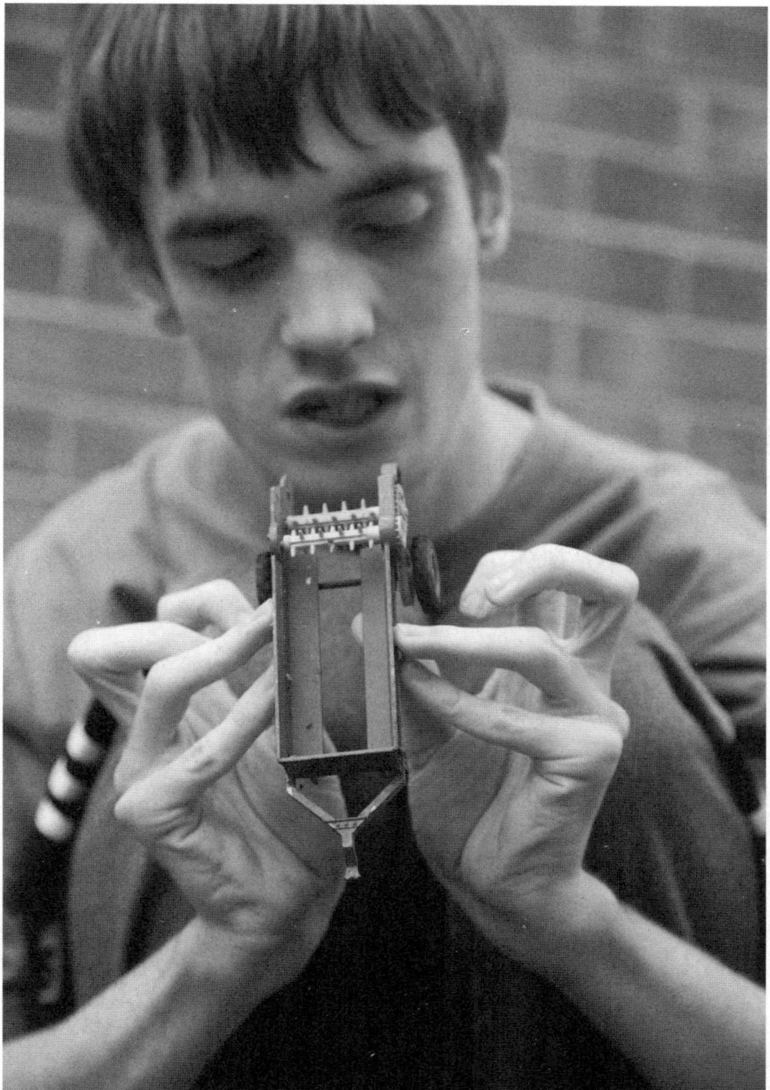

图16　当男孩看他的玩具车时，他看见各种通常会逃过我们眼睛的细节。似乎这些细节远比整个物体更重要。因此男孩不只是把玩具车当车玩，而且更感兴趣于它的零部件，特别是那些可以按、转、扭的部件

患有阿斯伯格综合征的查尔斯在一封电子邮件中写道："我有异乎寻常的强烈而狭窄的兴趣。这是个最贴切、最明显适用于我的特征。在十一岁到十八岁间，我对数学的确有极其强烈的兴趣。从四岁半到十三岁左右我对宝贝熊鲁柏非常感兴趣。从七岁左右到十三岁我对天文学非常感兴趣。最近几年我开始对学习外语特别感兴趣。"查尔斯天赋异禀。很典型的是，他描述的各种兴趣互不相关。它们突兀地开始和结束，但很明显持续相当长时间。

弱中央统合

为什么会被称为弱中央统合呢？它指的是追寻意义的通常比较强烈的动力。如果是强中央统合，会有预设的偏好，想要观察到整体而不是部分。我们观察画作是把它当作一个物体而不是一丛杂乱的线条；我们听见的是句子而不是一堆杂乱的词语。整体通常被称为格式塔（Gestalt），在德语中表示完全形态的意思。心理学家用它来解释，我们正常情况下为什么会倾向于观察到全局的整体而不是局部的部分。然而，只有在信息过量时才可能显示出这种偏好，而且你无法同时**兼顾整体和部分**。

情境是描述整体即格式塔及它与局部的关系的另一种方式。情境为局部赋予意义。在非常柔和的乐章中，某个单独音符可能听起来非常响亮。但同样的音符在吵闹的乐章中可能听起来很柔和。音高也同样如此。音高辨别力是指听出准确音高的能力，无论在什么样的情境中。令人称奇的是，大约30%的自闭症人士，即使未经专业音乐训练，也具有音高辨别力。

弱中央统合功能的意思是情境没有施加很多力量。在一
90 个特定情境内部，一点一画都能看出本来的样子——完全一

样——即使在另一种情境中它们看起来完全不同。在强中央统合当中，一个元素的意义会随情境而大幅改变，甚至有时会在另一种情境中完全认不出来是同一个元素。图17中所示的幻觉就是很好的例子。这里，中间的圆随着周围圆的情境而看起来或大或小。事实是它们的大小完全一样。如果你看它是大小一样，你就显示出弱中央统合。你不太容易被幻觉欺骗！显然，不被整体情境影响可能是大大的优点。有时，弱中央统合中的"弱"会被误解为"差"。其实大多数弱中央统合的测试都倾向于显示出好的或是优异的表现。

图17还展示出其他的视觉测试，自闭症人士在这些测试中表现良好。他们的共同点在于，他们青睐一种自动聚焦于细节的策略。这就是弗兰切斯卡·哈佩提及它的方式。关于这个观点，她已经做了非常多的理论和实验工作。例如，她表明，这种信息处理方式在相当数量的正常人群中也很典型，在自闭症孩子的大约一半的父亲和三分之一的母亲身上也是如此。

弗兰切斯卡·哈佩的实验室还设计了如下任务。把句子补充完整：你去打猎，带着一把刀和________。

如果填"叉子"，你则是弱中央统合的例子，在这个例子中指跟局部元素有联系。因为刀和叉经常连在一起说。同时你还忽视了句子的整体意思。假如填的内容类似于"捉住一头熊"，你就表现出强中央统合。另一个测试例子是："大海的味道是盐和________。"

你会不会填"胡椒"？这再次说明了弱中央统合的例子。如果填"鱼"之类的，你就把整个句子意思考虑在内，这是强中央统合的迹象。

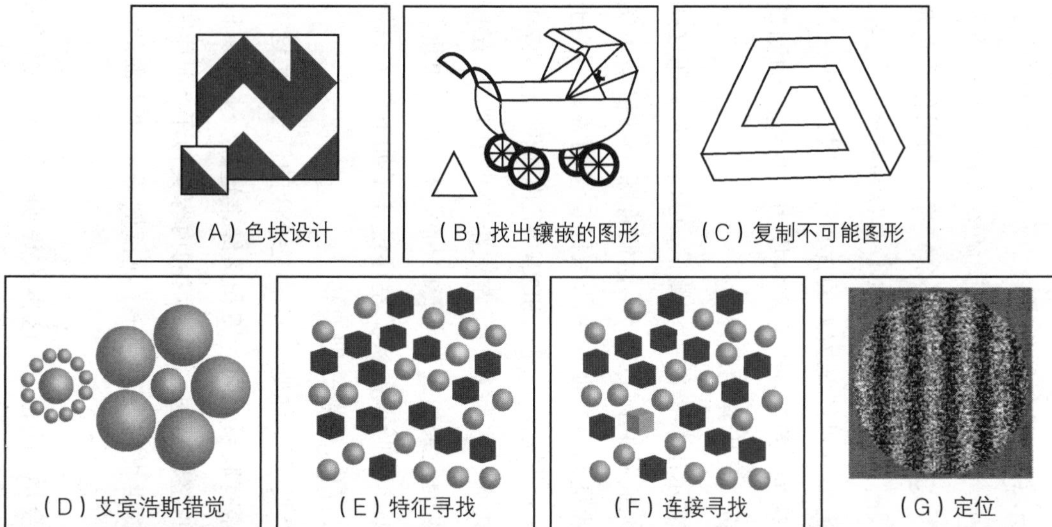

图17　自闭症谱系障碍人士通常表现优异的任务

根据第四大理论弱中央统合，自闭症人士观察世界的方式与众不同。注重细节的处理方式不仅是指视觉，还适用于听觉和语言。其他感官呢——比如触觉？这里一个有趣的现象是，很多自闭症人士据说对触觉过分敏感。拥有超敏感的触觉也许类似于拥有辨别音高的能力。

弱中央统合能不能解释天才技能？某种程度上是的。这种类型的信息处理方式，主要表现就是能够逐字逐句记住材料，即使并不了解内容。很明显其他因素也会有影响——例如练习。反复练习，甚至沉迷其中，对一个兴趣爱好非常狭窄的人来说，可不是件琐碎无聊的事。自闭症的典型表现之一是避免新奇事物，这一点也很有利于他们的反复练习。当大卫开始对印刷物着迷时，他读了几百遍《戴帽子的猫》。他已经记住了整本书，但还是反复读书上的每一页。他的文字阅读能力远远超越他的理解能力。

弱中央统合理论做了些很大胆的尝试，试图在自闭症智力的一些毫不相干的方面建立联系。它试图同时既能解释某些特殊天赋，也能解释某些认知缺陷。可能是因为试图用一种理论解释所有现象，它也就没有我们看过的前三大理论那么成功，而前三种理论只考察了缺陷。

对注意力的系统研究也许会澄清弱中央统合思想考察的现象。对细节和对整体的关注也许在本质上非常不同。当注意力从注重细小元素切换到注重大整体时，它发生了什么？反过来呢？研究表明，自闭症人士总体说来更倾向于近距离放大那些小元素，但不太能够缩小、拉远以注意到整体。

该理论的问题

研究者们已经尝试了很多任务，这些任务清楚表明自闭症人士察觉到格式塔并无困难。相反，他们有个强化的处理细节的机制。与弱中央统合相对应，这种理论叫作知觉促进增强理论。它提出，有一个独立的细节处理的**优先级**，而并非简单的格式塔处理的**次等级**的结果。系统化是另一种思想，它强调自闭症人士不只是看见微小的细节，而且热爱系统。正是这种对系统的热爱有可能解释一些天才技能，比如日历推算。

另一种批评认为，聚焦于细节的处理方式看起来只能适用于自闭症障碍的部分人而非所有人。如同我们从其他几大理论看到的一样，这个批评并不一定是致命的：没有哪个理论可能适用于自闭症谱系障碍的所有病例。必然有一些亚群体。

顶端的麻烦

是时候来介绍五大理论中的最后一个了——大脑中执行系统出错的理论。假如失去控制，你的行为就失去边界。**你陷进去了**而且很难走得出来。进一步说，你**被随机事件俘虏了**。你的行为基于冲动，而不是基于远见和规划。当正常路线行不通时，你不会停下来思考，去找到新奇的解决方案。另一方面，你**缺乏抑制**，表现出社交上不能接受的行为。如果执行系统崩溃，你在控制其他大脑系统时就会出现问题。这个理论试图解释自闭症人士在应对纷繁复杂的日常生活的压力时所遭遇的问题。有人可能认为这些问题只会出现在低功能病例身上。然而并非
94 如此，这些问题贻害很深，低功能和高功能人士都会受到妨害。

加里迫切地想找个女朋友，控制不住自己着迷地跟踪一个漂亮女人。有人告诉他这样不对。女人向警察投诉。他被严厉训斥，然而他的家人不相信他不会再犯。家人不得不严密监视他的行为。为什么他不能抑制自己完全正常的冲动呢？

神经心理学家们对这类问题并不陌生，大脑额叶受损的病人就会如此。额叶受损的病人会让人很困惑。在常规的智力测试中他们得分很高，但在日常生活中，他们会做糟糕的决定，不会做合适的规划，总体表现出无法使用智力来适应环境。

大脑的额叶的作用是做出高级的执行决定。在惯常行为不得体或是需要被打断或推翻的任何时候，这些执行决定都非常必要。这里列举一些日常生活中的典型问题，它们全部与高级控制系统受损有关。

陷进去了

有一个人叫作迈克尔·布拉斯特兰德，他给出的他儿子乔的例子用来说明这个问题再合适不过了。在很长一段时间里，他只吃一种牌子的乳清干酪和菠菜意大利面。即使很饿，他也会拒绝其他食物。他急于吃到这唯一的一种食物，有时甚至等不及煮熟。布拉斯特兰德还讲到乔会坚持一遍又一遍重复观看录像。这个故事令人苦恼的一面在于，乔在很多方面表现得像是一个上瘾者。他看录像有瘾。一旦得不到录像就无法安抚。然而，当他观看录像时，也没有很开心。乔的父母对他的极度渴求和他对新事物的极度排斥不知所措。幸运的是，乔长大后去了一所特殊学校，这些问题得到缓解。最终他学会了吃其他食 95
物，也学会了享受丰富多彩的活动。

被偶然事件俘虏

“每当鲍勃路过一所房子或者其他建筑，看见开着的门，他就要走进去探寻一番。无须赘言，这种行为经常会导致不愉快的冲突，但很明显，每次他都很惊讶，却从来没学会吸取教训。”这是通常被称为刺激驱动行为的一个例子。然而，我们完全正常的日常行为大多数都是刺激驱动的。与自闭症的不同之处在于，我们能让行为处于控制之下。对一个患自闭症的人来说，被某种以前触发过他们行为的东西偶然触发时，想要抑制某些行为需要付出巨大的努力。

缺乏抑制

马修的妈妈跟我讲，她每天处理垃圾时都要跟他有一场大战。马修不同意扔掉任何东西，连信封、包装纸都不能扔掉，更别提报纸和塑料袋了。这种问题有时在因中风导致的大脑额叶中部受损的病人身上也能看到。这些病人在导致损伤的事故之后开始搜集无用的东西。这并不意味着大脑的这些区域是搜集行为的基础。相反，这些区域是抑制搜集行为的基础，而这些病人在抑制方面有问题。在老鼠的大脑中——我们推测人类也是如此，存在着大脑深处区域，被称作皮质区，负责驱动获取和搜集行为。这种驱动在正常情况下是受控制的，能保持在合理的边界内。但这需要完好无损的额叶。

灾难地带

每当肯需要自己去买东西时就会感到压力很大。即使他列

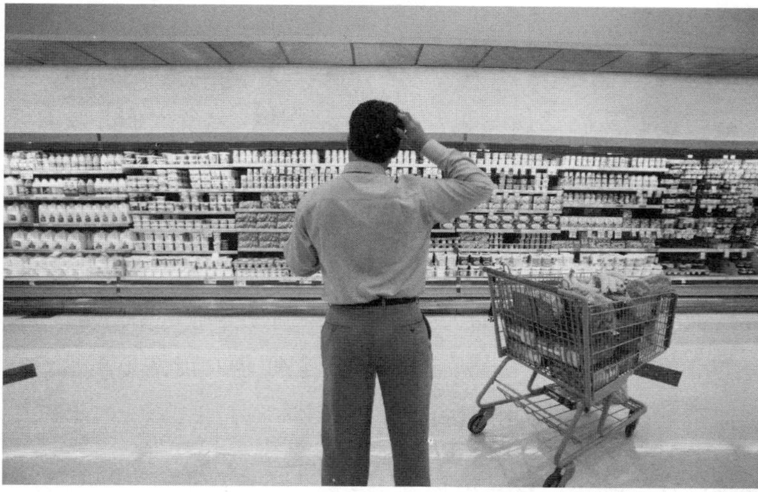

图18 在超市里执行功能被严重挑战，因为需要在预算范围内计划；需要抵制冲动型购物；需要抑制对特价的响应；需要为无货的物品找到替代。自闭症个体发现这种情形会造成巨大压力，但他们可以遵循确定步骤

了清单，尽量不被吸引去购买不必要的物品，还是会发生差错。有一天，他要买的牌子的麦片不在平常的货架上。他十分恐慌。肯不知道还能去问售货员会不会添货，还是它被放到了其他货架上。之前来这里时他被告知不能问售货员问题，麻烦他们。所以他就回家了，极其沮丧。这个例子相对温和，但能让我们略略理解为何许多需要灵活应对的日常生活事件成了主要的压力点。这种古怪的思维灵活性的缺乏，让他们的生活困难重重，即使对那些在其他方面能力很强的人也是如此。

由于额叶很大，所起的又是监管功能，额叶功能受损的效果既微妙又深远。当病人们不得不自发行动时，或是处于新奇或非结构化情境中时，会产生各种障碍。对肯来说也是如此。当熟悉的日常程序被打乱时，他就手足无措了。在这种情况下他 97

还会变得暴烈。

尽管足够多的证据暗示这些问题与糟糕的额叶功能有关，尽管与额叶功能受损的病人行为非常相似，至今人们并没有在自闭症的大脑额叶中找到缺陷。没有可见的解剖学上的异常。但额叶功能较弱可能是别处的问题造成的，或者是与其他大脑区域的联结问题造成的。研究仍在进行，想要确定当人们用扫描仪探寻时，自闭症中的大脑额叶在不同任务中是如何运作的。有一点已经很明确：虽然看上去非常健康，但功能并不正常。它们似乎是以不同方式组织的。

该理论的问题

执行功能异常的理论被广泛接受。进一步说，人们普遍认可大多数自闭症个体会出现日常生活的困难。但有个主要问题：这个理论非常宽泛，或许可以应用于几乎全部神经发育障碍上，而不仅仅是自闭症。

五大理论的关联：自上而下过程和自下而上过程之间对接失败

这一部分是关于尚未成熟的一些理论。所以你需要决定是愿意撸起袖子加入我接下来的部分，还是更愿意跳到下一章。

自上而下与自下而上——我喜欢这两个术语并频繁使用它们。我认为它们抓住了心智/大脑如何运作的非常重要的方面。这两种过程在我们觉知周围的世界时都必不可少，最重要的是
98 使我们的知觉有意义。以下是可能会发生的事情的简化版。

我们想象一下大脑分为两个系统。一个系统用来发送从外

部世界搜集来的货物，另一个系统用来控制下一步行动。粗略地说，大脑后部被发送过程占据着，而控制系统则在大脑前部。发送系统自下而上运作，而控制系统自上而下运作。两种系统都发挥作用，但必须协同运作。现在让我们假定在自闭症大脑中它们不合作了。假设是自下而上的系统运作正常，允许优先发送信息和优先执行不涉及控制系统的任何任务，但控制系统运作不太好。似乎对所有五大理论都是如此。

当我在一次会议上陈述此理论时，一位阿斯伯格综合征人士站起来说，他要写信给我。他的短信如下："经验告诉我从不该试图理解任何事情。那只对神经正常的人有用，但你需要自上而下地思考来让它运作。还是分析和计算对我们更有用。"他总算是理解我了：他把自上而下的控制比拟为理解，把自下而上的发送比拟为分析和计算。

自上而下的系统究竟重要在什么地方？已有众多来自知觉神经科学的证据表明，对于自下而上进入大脑的信息，大脑以自上而下的信息调制方式运作。并不是进入大脑的所有信息都拥有同等的价值。自上而下的控制系统需要把好的和坏的分别归类拣出来，再把这一点传达给发送系统。它发送信号，导致有用的信息被增强，无用的信息被压制。自上而下的系统控制发送系统的一种方式是通过它预先的期待。这些期待受文化浸染， 99
受我们与他人的社会关系影响。这就产生了前面三种理论。

厨师和食客

让我们想象有一位非常挑剔的食客，坐在楼上餐厅，还有一位异常忙碌的厨师，在楼下马不停蹄地忙着。厨师提供给楼上的大多数食物都被拒绝了，食客认为值得食用的只有挑剔的一小口。食客有些特别偏好，自然希望能影响厨师只使用他最喜爱的原材料。他让厨师知道，如果吃到新鲜的最优质的白芦笋，他总会开心。然而厨师需要用市场能提供的原料做菜。

食客如何跟厨师沟通？当然是通过服务员。服务员工作难做。他不得不向厨师传达食客的过分要求。他也不得不向食客传达一点厨房里的现实情况。他希望至少有时食客的偏好能匹配厨师当天的专长。

服务员不得不在两种关注点间耍点手段，一边是厨师的典型关注，一边是食客的典型关注。厨师的注意力完全来自他从市场上获取的食材。例如，去市场时他会抵挡不住一篮篮汁多鲜美的草莓的诱惑。无论如何他都会被吸引住。然而，进入厨师法眼的有诱惑力的食材总有很多。随后，这些食材自动被准备好，按各自的方式：切碎、切丁、削皮、蒸煮、烘烤、白煮或是煎炒。

而另一方面，食客的关注点是从内部产生的。他从不去市场，但用记忆和从其他食客处获得的知识来要求特别的、通常还
100 是新奇的食物。举个例子。另一位食客打电话给我们这位食客，诱使他点风靡一时的鸭蛋。服务员立刻行动，告诉厨师。当食客想要煎鸭蛋时，厨师必须停止使用鸡蛋，识别出鸭蛋。

有时，双方共事良好。当厨师给出食客想要的煎蛋时，食客的喜悦溢于言表。有时自上而下的关注点与自下而上的关注点互相较劲。食客大叫要芦笋，而厨师正忙着灭厨房里的火。在这种情况下，食客得不到想要的。然而，他现在可以订一个更加高效的灭火器。

这则寓言解释的是大脑的控制和发送系统的互动。两者中哪一个都不比另一个更重要。最后一个例子表明，控制系统不能够改写发送系统中的紧急情况。然而，它可以采取行动阻止紧急情况的再次发生。我的假设是，在自闭症中这两种大脑系统的互动运作不好。这究竟是谁的过错，漠然的食客，热心过头的厨师，还是莫名其妙的服务员？他们都有可能，但我个人倾向于认为是食客的错。

自上而下的调节

在视觉观察的自上而下的控制中，大脑里究竟发生了什么？大脑影像实验给了我们一些线索。在这个实验中，人们事先被告知他们的注意力要集中在屏幕上。屏幕上一对对图片飞快闪过。重要的是，受试者只能看见它们，也只在这时他们才被事先告知看哪里。现在图片是脸部或者房屋。这个选择很聪明，因为看房屋和看脸部的大脑活动区域在不同地方。这是从其他实验已知的。在这个实验中，当闪过房屋或者脸部时，这些 101
大脑区域确实变得活跃了。并且，当受试者注意力被引导至它们一会儿将要出现的位置时——通过测试人员提示——这些区域变得更活跃。换句话说，自上而下的注意力增强了大脑活动。自闭症人士也参加了一模一样的测试并接受大脑扫描。他们表现出少得多的活跃性的提升。这个实验直接证明，在自闭症大脑层面，缺乏自上而下的调节。

难以调节注意力的人更可能被外部刺激物抓住注意力。同时，他们又发现很难强行拉走自己的注意力。这可能就是为什么乔一直都吃同样的食物，为什么爱德华的兴趣狭窄而受限，以及为什么大卫有着惊人但不求甚解的记忆力的原因。

缺席的食客

这其实是个相当冒险的理论——我把这部分写出来仅仅是因为我希望能找到这个问题的答案：在自上而下过程中这个“上”究竟是什么？我即刻的简短回答是，自上而下中的“上”其实是**自我**。这个自我其实就是我先前故事里提到的食客。食客有特定的偏好和期待，永远影响着从厨房给他呈上来的东西。所以自我是有偏好的，会影响大脑如何处理信息。食客挑选他希望尝试的食物。自我决定对什么感兴趣，对什么没兴趣。缺席的自我是自下而上和自上而下的处理失衡的特征之一。

假如食客缺席，人们会以为厨师不再受到上层的奇奇怪怪要求的阻碍，将能够完全利用手头的食材，烹制出最美味的饭菜，完全能做出他最擅长的，用他独特的切碎、切丁、削皮、蒸煮、烘烤、白煮或是煎炒技巧。这是理解天才技能的一种方式。

但其中难道没有问题吗？乔坚持吃完全一样的某种食物是怎么回事？这难道不是表明他有非常强烈的自我？或者用比喻的意义来说，是一个有着强烈预先设定的期待的食客？我不认为如此。毕竟，如父亲迈克尔·布拉斯特兰德所描述的，乔的这种期待毫无理性。回应也是冥顽不化的刻板。对我来说，这意味着简单的关联学习或工具性情形。这里命令链的顶端是孤立但根深蒂固的对刺激物的回应，这个刺激物曾经让他满足过。这还是厨师在孤军奋战，做他最擅长的食物。但没有目的，因为上层没有食客。

这里我们需要回忆食客的另一个特征，他的社交兴趣以及与其他食客交流的能力。他想吃什么，并不只是随意做出决定，而是根据目前流行什么来做决定。我们可以想象一个食客并未缺席很多，但他不跟其他食客交流。

一些初步结论

在本章中，自闭症的无社交特征被放到聚光灯下。这既有优势也有弱点。第四大理论叫作弱中央统合，它使我们赞叹自闭症人士的优势，也使我们信任他们的特殊天分。第五大理论通常被称为执行功能失调，它关注他们在应对日常生活时面临的无尽困难。

我对比了大脑中一个系统的优势——和信息发送有关，与另一系统的弱点——和信息控制有关。有证据表明，大脑的控制系统有弱点，但发送系统有优势。 103

在本章的最后一部分，我努力推测在自上而下和自下而上过程中有一种失衡。但还有很多问题。为什么自闭症人士的表现方式各异呢？为什么他们不能分享其他人的社交社会和物理社会？我认为应该归咎于大脑的自上而下的控制系统，问题出在一个缺失的自我，至少是一个缺乏与其他社交个体进行正常互动的自我。

最终会不会有一种令人满意的理论形成，来解释自闭症典型的深陷沉迷和缺乏灵活性的特征？也许。那个缺失的自我的概念，能不能抓住自闭症典型的自上而下的控制和自下而上的发送之间的失衡？可能，也只是可能而已。 104

第七章

从理论到实践

三个盒子的游戏

在探索自闭症的过程中，黛安娜调查了很多事实，看见了自闭症的多面性，学习了那些试图深入到自闭症人士思维里的心理学实验。这些加起来能得到什么？有没有一个大一统的理论呢？很不幸，还没有。自闭症障碍的各种症状相去甚远，纷繁复杂，尚无令人满意的单一描述出现。

然而，黛安娜想要梳理好她已经学习到的东西。她仍然深深为之着迷，思索着是否应该自己做点关于自闭症的研究。以她自然科学方面的背景，她有很好的知识储备来学习神经科学的必要技巧。把她现在所知的都糅合起来，这主意不错。这样她就能看出还缺失什么，以及在未来还需要做哪些事来找出更加完善的自闭症成因。

这里给她一点帮助。首先，黛安娜必须梳理一下她已有的许多知识碎片。通过简单的小诀窍，可以给她的梳理过程提供莫大帮助：把知识碎片放进三个盒子里。三个盒子分别是：**生物学**、**思维**和**行为**。每个盒子对应一种特别的知识：生物学盒子里是目前已搜集到的关于大脑和基因的知识；思维盒子里是从有关思维的实验研究中获得的结论；行为盒子里是行为方面广为接受的事实。在每个盒子中，她可以把她所了解的事情列出来。 105

这个梳理操作中引人注目的一点是，思维盒子是另两个盒子之间的核心关联。在行为盒子里，黛安娜有一系列自闭症标志和症状，形式多样，变化多端。第一章和第二章囊括了很多这些事实。在生物学盒子里，她有一系列事实，有些事实在第三章和第四章中有所呈现。

思维的盒子装满了在以上两章讨论的各种理论。这里我们论述理论，而非罗列事实，这无可厚非。这些理论都经过各种测试，绝非空穴来风。这些理论我个人敢打赌能历经时间考验，它们背后都有深厚的实验研究支持。这些特征的神经学基础已有强烈的暗示，但只是暗示而已。黛安娜很心动，想去亲自做点这些工作。

我们在生物学的盒子里找到什么

对于自闭症的成因，黛安娜已经列出长长的影响因素：发育不稳定性、遗传倾向性、变异、环境风险因素、概率和事故。这些不同的可能性不互相排斥，也不互相孤立。相反，它们可能结合起来，导致自闭症谱系障碍的多样性。然而，看起来很难在基因层面辨别不同的成因。不同的成因可能会最终影响一条同样的路径，导致相似的大脑思维异常，以及相似的迹象和症状。

对自闭症大脑我们还知之甚少。自闭症儿童有更大的大脑，但不是出生时就如此，而是在一岁之后被观察到有段快速增长期，而在大约八岁之后有所下降。这个事实可能与神经联结
106 的此消彼长有关：先是神经联结的大量增生，随后是猛烈地修剪。这些极度复杂和动态过程中的干扰因素，可能是众多不同成因的最终共同路径。

我们在行为学的盒子里找到什么

黛安娜回忆起，自闭症目前是通过行为表现确诊的。这里她列出了自闭症的核心特征，及其他常见特征，比如过度敏感和言语重复。行为特征是有问题的，因为它们随着年龄、能力，以及其他许多因素的不同而不同，这些因素导致的不同并不是隐藏情形的一部分。并没有一套自闭症独一无二的行为，如果是那样，就能清楚无疑地确诊自闭症了。两个孩子，即便他们的自闭症是由相同的生物学因素引起的，也可能看起来互不相同。每个孩子都会表现出不同的行为方式。它取决于很多因素，他们自身的内部资源、他们的教育程度，以及从外部世界得到的支持。我们很欣慰地得知，支撑性的教育环境会产生广泛的影响。它甚至可以掩盖现存的问题。这些影响具体是如何运作的？我们仍不清楚。

我们在思维的盒子里找到什么

很明显，五大理论应该放在思维的盒子里。这些理论能够把行为盒子里的点点滴滴拼凑起来，尽管那些点滴原先看起来互不相关。黛安娜立刻就明白，如果她进一步搜寻，还能发现

更多的类似理论。但五个理论是不错的开始。思维的盒子会很有用，因为她可以把以后听到的关于自闭症的所有思想和理论——甚至她自己创造出来的——都临时倾倒在此。重要的是，一旦承认这些理论，必须有一些审查，并需要严格的测试。缺乏社交驱动的理论令人信服，心智化的理论有点奇怪，碎镜理论很新奇，它们都要解释自闭症印记的不同方面，此印记即交互性社交互动的缺乏。弱中央统合理论试图解释天才技能及整体 107
看待世界的不同方式。弱执行功能理论试图解释自闭症的所有日常困难。总而言之，五大理论一起让自闭症的很多令人费解的现象变得有意义。进一步说，它们为有可能出错的内在神经机制提供了研究线索。

这些盒子如何拼装

令人沮丧的是，究竟是什么导致自闭症这个问题还没有答案。风险因素非常多，遗传的、环境的都有。这些因素的效果对于思维和对于大脑是一样的。最终受到影响的可能是一条共同的大脑/思维路径。其中的意味非常重要。即使自闭症的成因变化多端，就导致的行为类型而言，它们却有其共同特性。这是一种认知表现型。也许会有不止一种共同路径，不止一种认知表现型。如果自闭症谱系的不同亚群体被诊断出来，情况可能就是这样。

假如这五大理论的每一个都被定义为一种认知表现型呢？基本上你可以想象一种认知表现型来封装某个理论。可能这种划分会让探究自闭症成因更简单点。有没有可能存在五种类型的自闭症？有可能。但还有一种可能性。五大理论指出的错误会被全部混合在一起，就像蛋糕原料一样。原料以不同的数量被加进去，有些原料还是可选的。可以想象不同的混合方法将会呈现出自闭症谱系的不同的点。

我们再次以心智化为例。一种心智化的错误是否就能定义自闭症谱系的一个亚群体？什么类型的**自闭**行为是它能解释的？它能够解释其核心特征，即不能够参与进真正的交互式社交互动和交流。这包含了一大类行为，我们在早先章节已经谈
108 及过。它适合我们三个例子的每一个，尽管大卫、加里和爱德华在自闭症谱系当中处于相当不同的位置。

在每个例子中他们的能力各不相同，他们所受教育和得到的帮助也完全不同，那又如何辨别他们的心智化错误呢？你需要一系列的测试。而这些测试还不存在。这些测试必须提供选择，难度适中；测试必须可靠且必须最终与实际生活行为相联系。单个病例原则上可以用大脑成像来测试。既然大脑的心智化系统是孤立的，在这个系统中功能异常应该可见。已有的结论表明，这个系统各部分之间的联结应该较弱。

我们来看另外一个例子。大卫、加里和爱德华表现出弱中央统合的一种认知表现型吗？这个表现型代表了一些人，他们偏好将注意力集中在细节上，且不容易分心。这里又需要一系列的测试——难度适中程度、可靠度和有效度的测试。这些测试很可能包括注意力测试和智力测试，毕竟，弱中央统合理论的目标之一是解释智力的不均衡模式。我们可能怀疑加里没有这种表现型——他并没有出色的能力，也没有狭窄的兴趣——但大卫很可能有。比如，他在拼图游戏中表现出色。对爱德华来说，在他最好和最差的表现当中我们也会发现巨大的差异。特

征大脑激活模式的测试还要寄望于未来。人们也许预计他们会表现出联结错误。这可能意味着大脑较远区域的联结太少，而在邻近区域的联结过多。可以用个交通的类比：没有大的高速公路，但有大量的本地小路。

对黛安娜来说，这些盒子开始连贯起来。联结错误有可能是造成缺乏心智化、缺乏社交驱动、碎镜系统、弱中央统合和自 109
上而下的控制困难的原因。

大脑中的联结和联结错误

让我们假设在自闭症大脑中，线条交错。例如，正常情况下，当人们解读思维时，大脑的若干部分即刻活跃起来，同步工作。在自闭症中看起来并非如此。可能在解读思维的大脑部分的联结之所以很弱，完全是因为在这些相对遥远的区域高速公路的联结太少，有的区域在大脑中部，有的在边上，有的在后部。

自闭症是一种神经发育障碍，它看起来是由大脑发育的混乱引起的。这一点现在对黛安娜能说得通了。但她需要在论证中更进一步。混乱可能是由于特定神经联结缺乏修剪。她不得不考虑另一个问题：为什么自闭症只会从生命中的第二年才明显起来？她想知道在一到两岁之间大脑的哪种联结发生了增生？我只能做个猜测，令人信服的结果应该是控制系统的各种联结。从动物大脑可视部分的运转我们知道，发送系统的自下而上的联结是准备好、等待着的，远在控制系统的自上而下的联结成熟之前。

让我们假设正是自上而下的联结先增生而后被修剪。有可能在自闭症当中，恰恰是这些联结没有在恰当的时机被修剪。

如果是这样，将能一举解释三件事情：发送系统出色的知觉能力；失速的控制系统的受限调制能力；以及第二年自闭症症状
110 的出现。它还可能同时解释在一岁后自闭症大脑的突增。

黛安娜决定，好的研究项目是尝试操控一个联结错误的大脑，比如在一只老鼠身上进行实验。它是如何起作用的？她将如何测试老鼠？它的能力应该不均匀分布。它应该是某些任务完成良好，而另一些任务完成不好，特别是那些需要自上而下控制的任务，以及那些需要精细社交感的任务。

黛安娜已经决定来应对这个问题，我深感欣慰。任务类型正确的话，应该有可能显示大脑中有系统在正常情况下共同工作，但在自闭症大脑中联结更弱。我相信最终自上而下的这个“上”必然被辨别出来，它正是负责控制的部分。我自己已经想过，这是不是“自我”的一种形式。这个自我在自闭症中是缺席的吗？这会揭示自闭症这个词的深层含义吗？毕竟自闭症（autism）这个词来源于希腊语中表示自我的词*autos*。我还给不了答案。然而，我满怀希望地期待迎来下一波实验研究。

自闭症谱系概念的冲突分歧

在写作这本书的过程中，我一直强烈地意识到使用例子时的冲突，例子有时是严重的经典自闭症病例，有时是非常高功能的病例以及阿斯伯格综合征。儿童和成人病例的例子也有差距。关于患上自闭症是什么感觉的那些轶事，全部来自高功能的成人。因此有一种危险，即自闭症谱系障碍的观点很大程度上向谱系的这个部分倾斜。这部分人被称作温和的自闭症并不一定正确，因为这些人有障碍。他们只是有时被补偿行为掩盖

起来一点点而已。另一方面，他们的自闭症特征与经典病例相比的确要温和一些。111

在我已经描述的研究中，实验通常依赖那些正常或高智力水平的参与者，因为那些技术和任务都对受试者要求很高。这些实验已经揭示了一些振奋人心的结果，大量描述这些实验，我问心无愧。当我记起我了解的经典病例，看起来所有五大理论都能派上用场来解释其行为，这些理论似乎能同时应用。但当我研究高功能病例时就不一样了。这时我的感觉是对具体个人的病例来说，部分而不是全部五大理论可以用来解释他们的困难。

所有这些使我思考，在未来研究中，人们可以对严重自闭症提出单独的问题，严重自闭症通常伴随着智力障碍，而温和的自闭症形式通常没有智力障碍。把一个群体的研究成果推广到另一个群体似乎不大可能，因此很明显有必要单独对待这些亚群体。我们就从那些高智商的开始吧。

在整本书中我们有过大量机会来看特殊人群的例子，他们有自闭症状况但能跟我们讲述他们的经历。坦普·葛兰汀就是这样的人。她作为作家、演讲家和动物行为的研究者而广受褒奖。坦普·葛兰汀的网站展示了她许多令人惊叹的才能。她能说出来高功能自闭症意味着什么，她强调思维方式的某些优势，对她来说她的思维方式是视觉思维。她对能够自立很满意，也显示了即使没有参与交互式交流，也可以过上充实、实现自我的人生。坦普·葛兰汀并不是唯一把她的生活、她的兴趣和心路历程写出来的自闭症人士。现在有很多书，那些极富才华的作者从第一人称的角度来揭露患有自闭症究竟是什么样。112

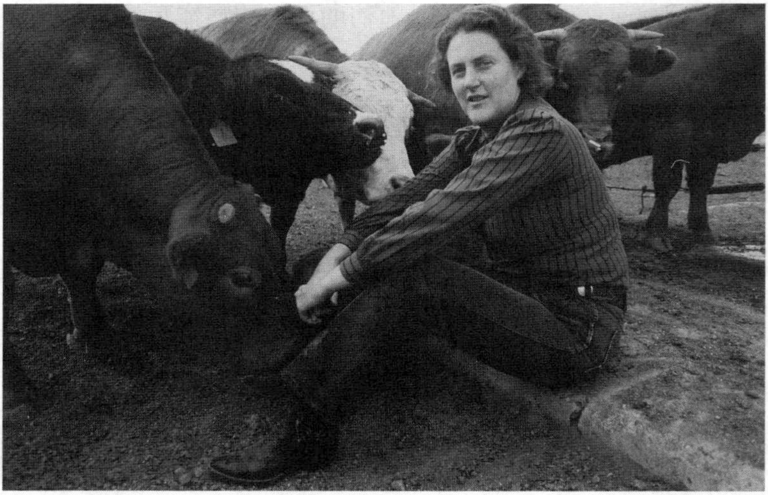

图19　坦普·葛兰汀是自闭症的杰出人士的代言人。她写过几本书，讲述自闭症究竟是什么样。她设计了牲畜设备，并对动物有特殊的热爱。她在《翻译动物：利用自闭症之谜解码动物行为》（纽约：斯克里布纳出版社2005年版）一书里写了这一切

假如你遇到坦普·葛兰汀这种人

这有点像遇到一个明星。更有可能的是你会碰到像爱德华这样的人，他的事例我们已经反复提及。你有可能**不会**立刻注意到爱德华有什么“不同”。然而，对爱德华来说，看上去正常和表现正常是付出了巨大努力的。你可能很惊奇，当你只是随意聊天时，他非常焦虑甚至快要晕厥。在他的思想中，任何事都可能发生。你可能突然变得有敌意；你可能突然发出了不合理的要求。普通人允许这样的事发生，只需耐心聆听，做出鼓励性的评论。作为规则，你的直接和坚定会有回报。爱德华很可能不会将礼貌的暗示当作停止谈论鸟蛋的信号。假如幸运的话，

爱德华将会在研究机构找到一份工作。他甚至可能在数学的某个领域做出重大发现。

要当心。被诊断为自闭症的一些高功能人士有可能其实并不属于自闭症谱系，而是有其他某种性格问题。当然他们会让你相信他们患上了阿斯伯格综合征。但你要能看出圈套的危险。要想跳出这个圈套，努力了解自闭症谱系的边界很有必要。

假如你遇到某人既有自闭症又有智力障碍

当你遇见四十岁的西尔维娅时，异样的事情会使你震惊。你会立刻知道她有“特殊需要”。西尔维娅是经典的自闭症女孩，表现淡漠疏离，坚持一成不变。她有天赋也有困难。她在一个特殊学校表现不错，不幸的是，在青春期她的行为问题更严重了。她还患了癫痫。随着体力增强，她不理解东西时就会沮丧，导致破坏东西，伤害他人和自己。她现在需要持续监视。对于自闭症只是不同而不是障碍这种说法，她的家人连理解的时间都没有。他们感觉这种说法简直是残忍的嘲讽。毫无疑问，自闭症已经严重损害西尔维娅的生活。但我们是否应该伤心、哀叹她的命运？未必。西尔维娅只是很模糊地意识到自己的问题，而且她和任何一个生活在有爱的环境里的人一样快乐。

加里又如何呢？你当然知道他有点古怪。你可能对他的邋遢外表和粗野行为退避三舍。你遇见他时，很可能认为他是个流浪汉。他经常嘟囔着抱怨没有得到公正的机会，但其实，只要让他安静下来他还是相当满足的。自从加入阿斯伯格综合征互助组，他已经找到相处时能感觉舒服的人、找到可以做朋友的人了。他甚至还在互助组里找到了个女朋友。他可能永远找不到

工作，当他不能再住家里时，他将会依赖社工服务来安排住处和
114 提供帮助。

患有自闭症谱系障碍需要花费多少？

健康经济学家还真算出来照顾一位具有自闭症谱系状况的人一辈子需要花费多少。在英国，一位自闭症高功能人士据估算要花费290万英镑，而低功能人士一生则需要470万英镑。现在大多数资金都花在生活辅助上。然而，很多情况还达不到理想的生活所需。社会服务和特殊教育长期缺乏资金，还很容易把更多资金花费在促进和提高它们的工作上。

但估算经济负担是一回事，人工成本又是一回事，而且完全不可能估算。很明显，减轻自闭症造成的负担势在必行。

教育和康复

分别教育高功能和低功能孩子的实践指导已有很多。幸运的是，对严重自闭症的孩子也有了有效的教育项目。我曾提过应用行为分析。在这里，合适的技巧和行为是通过学习理论原则教授的。音乐疗法和艺术疗法也都有其益处。言语疗法可以极大帮助提高发音和使用语言。各种疗法都不是听上去那么简单，因此需要训练有素的治疗师。通常还需要好几项技巧的结合才行。一个有天分又投入的老师或是父母会带来很大改变，这同时也意味着，我们并不真正知道神奇成分究竟是什么。

所用的技巧中有些含有非常高强度的社交情感互动和游
115 戏。例如，有一种比生活更夸张的互动，为增强这种互动，他们像母亲们对婴儿那样，使用变调的声音和面部表情。对稍大的

孩子和青少年，社交技能训练很受欢迎，效果明显。引人入胜的资料随处可得，例如有些动画片和电影非常清晰地呈现着情感的表达。

一个例子是《托马斯小火车》。这是一本颇受孩子们欢迎的书，而且看起来是自闭症孩子们的最爱。家长们认为，小火车头们清晰的面部表情和简单的社交互动故事解释了诸如合作、 116
竞争、骄傲、焦虑及嫉妒，看上去非常适合作为教学辅助。“小火车们的名字是他在会叫妈妈爸爸之前就会念的第一批单词。”为

图20　W. V. 奥德里为孩子们写的小火车系列童书。《托马斯小火车》在1946年问世，一直以来享誉世界。自闭症孩子们被火车头的图片吸引，它们有独特的个性和传神的表情，孩子们能通过故事学习社交信号

数不少的家长如是描述。

我们很容易访问剑桥自闭症研究中心的网站，它就是用了小火车的创意，起名叫“运输者”。这些改编过的故事里的主人公，被用来辅助教授社交技巧和社交信号。这些主人公展现了清楚、简化的情感表达。设计简洁，故事简单，这似乎才能巩固学习，寓教于乐。

我们需要什么样的教学和社交帮助？

决定以后人生的教育、工作和住房，并非一劳永逸的事情。在讨论自闭症人士的需求和权利时，人们常感困惑，因为自闭症谱系极为宽广。不可能做出适用于所有人的普遍规定。他们需要的服务多种多样，数目庞大。

教育方面也是如此。有关特殊需求学校和融合教育的讨论从未停止过。家长们可能很希望让他们的孩子上到主流学校，认为这才是他们孩子学会适应并学习社交技能的地方，这纯粹是出于与其他孩子相处的需要。如果与别的孩子在一起就能学会社交就好了！相反，大多数自闭症孩子如果在特殊小组或特殊学校中，接受一位专业教师在平静且高度结构化的环境里的教学，才更有可能获益。但对这一点并没有达成共识，辩论仍将持续。自
117 闭症的表现太多样，给每个孩子制订单独计划可能更合理。

药物治疗

针对自闭症的药物治疗并不存在。然而，伴随症状，如癫痫、高度焦虑或抑郁等可以通过用药来控制。对自闭症来说，如正常发育一样，也很有必要警惕各种医疗情形。很多病症发生

在自闭症孩子身上的可能性异常地高，例如胃黏膜炎症和过敏反应。很多这类病症是可以治愈的。

如果患有胃黏膜炎症但并不知道如何表达，那么孩子可能会表现出一系列的行为问题，比如咬人、尖叫。如果炎症能用恰当的药物治疗，孩子会安静、快乐得多，即使交流的深层问题并没有消失。

食疗干预有些狂热的支持者。对食物过敏的糟糕症状也可能对行为有影响，因此考虑过敏的影响很有意义。然而，只有部分自闭症孩子可能会出现这样的过敏。

骗子们

只要存在治愈自闭症的需求，就总会有人说他们能提供治愈方法。我们自然不会说自闭症像是肺结核一样的疾病，多亏现代药物才能治愈。如我们在第四章所讨论的，自闭症很大程度是一种基于基因的疾病，行为表现形式如彩虹般有各个不同的侧面。自闭症也并非总是一种障碍，并非总是负担。对这些病例来说，想要治愈他们显然很荒谬。但对以残障为主的那些病例来说，希望能减轻或预防并不荒谬。然而，我们还没有恰当的知识来完成。任何承诺有捷径的人，不管是通过特殊饮食补 118
充还是什么养生法，都有骗子的嫌疑。幸运的是，已经有一些网站，警告大家注意有潜在危险的以及未经验证的治疗方案。

假如你是父母、照料者，或是教师，有一点值得了解。发育是非常强大的力量。随着时间推移，在行为、社交技能和语言上不断进步是顺理成章的事。对自闭症孩子来说也是如此。这些进步的发生可能并不需要做特别的事情，只需在正常层面或高于正常水平加以照料和支持即可。有可能教育项目在可期待的进步之上能产生显著的进步。然而，评估这些项目极其困难。只有好的做法，但没有达成共识的最佳做法。

压力

不会交流、不能参与交互式交流，还有着刻板的行为方式和过于沉迷的倾向，要照顾这样的孩子，对任何家庭来说很明显都是沉重的负担。甚至对那些拥有丰富物质资源的家庭，即使拥有能提供服务的社区网络，仍是项十分艰巨的工作。你还可以想想自闭症孩子的兄弟姐妹们。

只要你不责怪他们使用一些手段去控制紧张局面，父母们就很感谢你了。当你看见一家人挣扎着坐飞机旅行，而他们的自闭症孩子非常执著地要喝饮料，请同情一下他们。是的，他们极可能已经想过给他饮料喝了！但不行，并非他们冷酷也并非他们无能。毫无疑问他们根据以往经验已经深知，必须无视这种反复的要求。

对这样的家庭来说，主要压力并不是“其他人怎么想”。他
119 们可能对别人的皱眉和“你不该这么做”的暗示已经免疫。主要压力完全来自关于自闭症的尚无答案的问题。连这样的情形是什么原因导致的都不知道，多令人沮丧。假如我们能知道病因，我相信家长们的态度将会从迷茫走向更好的应对和寻求被更多人接受。很多人可以被接受，很多人能有积极的前景，甚至得到幸福。但这不是唯一标准。

对自闭症个体的压力，其后果很可能比健康人更糟糕。如能避免，事情就能令人愉快地朝着好的方向发展。反之，如果有

行为的突然恶化，去找找可能导致的压力。所以对那些与自闭症人士有日常接触的人，最实际的实践建议通常也就是这样：努力找出压力源，然后消除压力源。压力源可能不明显。比如，可能只是一种非结构化的情形，比如不得不决定要吃什么的时候。

你无须害怕自闭症人士。他们与众不同，但正如马克·哈登小说里的主人公克里斯托弗一样，他们也很努力表现得像其他任何人一样。他们有可能做事夸张，有可能惹恼旁人，比如在尴尬的时间问奇怪的问题。假如从基础研究中获得了一些基本知识和理解，你有可能处理得更好。你不需要寻求关于该说什么、该做什么的特别建议，这永远不会切合具体的人或具体的场景；你可以针对一个问题自己构思，然后全面考虑。

本书传达的信息是，科学研究已经回答了关于自闭症令人困惑的部分问题，未来还将回答尚未解决的许多问题。为自闭症人士选择合适的教育和照料没有捷径。非常重要的是，研究处在相当基础的层面，特别是在大脑和思维层面。 120

我们还需要了解更多的事情

自闭症之谜仍在召唤我们去解决。在本书中的许多地方，我已经暗示了我们无知的黑点。不管怎样，我们需要更多了解思维/大脑是如何运作的。例如，经历共情时、用眼神接触时、认出人脸时，简而言之，当我们参与进和他人的社会交流时，大脑里究竟发生了什么？我们需要知道关于思维/大脑的更多机制，这些机制使我们能够意识到自我，意识到我们与他人的关系。也许，最最诱惑人的是，我们需要找到天才禀赋的秘密。

然而，我们也可以把这些无知的黑点看作位于尚未开发的新大陆上的白点。各种探险家，特别是那些把心理学实验和神经科学的技术结合起来的人，以及能够联手细胞生物学家和遗传学家一起工作的人，将会填补地图空白，他们带回的答案预示着丰厚回报。这些答案不仅让我们能够更好地理解自闭症人士，还能让我们了解所有人为什么是现在的样子。

对黛安娜，我的建议是她不该惧怕创造出其他重大理论，她可以努力批判性地仔细阅读本书中所述的各大理论。关于扩大知识的疆界，没什么比尝试初看有点疯狂的理论更好的方式
121 了——只要这些方式能经受实验的检验。

索　引

（条目后的数字为原书页码，见本书边码）

A

B

C

D

E

F

G

H

I

J

K

L

M

N

O

P

Uta Frith

AUTISM

A Very Short Introduction

Contents

Acknowledgements

I thought this short introduction would be quick and easy to write. How wrong! It was a long, slow and sometimes uncomfortable process. It made me revisit my past and review different ideas about autism, having to make selections as well as omissions. It made me realize that there are rather few solid facts about autism. Instead, I have selected what I consider good bets about the results of still ongoing research. I am hopeful that the studies I have picked will stand the test of time.

Given these difficulties it was imperative that I had knowledgeable reviewers. I was very fortunate to count Chris Frith, Francesca Happé, and Sarah White among them. They gave invaluable advice and critically important suggestions for improvement. They did not discourage me from including some more speculative thoughts.

I would also like to thank my most constant and constructive critics, Alex and Martin Frith. Alex edited most of the chapters in a sensitive and accomplished manner. My friend, Heide Grieve, as always gave excellent advice. I am deeply grateful to Chris, Franky and Sarah for helping me to decide what should be included in this introduction to autism and what could be left out. This book belongs to them.

Aarhus, 24 January 2008

List of illustrations

The publisher and the author apologize for any errors or omissions in the above list. If contacted they will be pleased to rectify these at the earliest opportunity.

Chapter 1
The autism spectrum

Is it autism?

Imagine a young mother and her baby. She adores him, and he is gorgeous. But, deep down Diane can't help worrying just occasionally, whether Mickey will grow up a normal happy boy. How could she tell if he has autism, for example? There is so much about autism in the news. Almost one in a hundred children born are autistic with five times as many boys as girls. An autistic child conjures up all sorts of scenarios, most of them bleak. And what are the first signs of autism? Is it significant that Mickey cries a lot, doesn't sleep much and is not easily calmed? Lots of babies are like that, Diane's mother says. She worries, however, that Mickey does not always turn around when she calls him from across the room.

When Diane started to read about autism she found the information quite unsettling. She read that some children are very delayed in their general development. Then there were some children who gave no cause for concern at all until well into their second year of life. One child never spoke; another was actually a little genius. Diane, like many people who are starting to find out about autism, is perplexed, but also intrigued.

The enigma of autism

When I first started to study autism as a young student in London in the 1960s I too was perplexed and intrigued. More than that, I was utterly fascinated as well as puzzled by the children I saw at London's Maudsley Hospital, where I trained to be a clinical psychologist. Because of this fascination I never worked as a clinical psychologist, but became a research scientist instead. But of course, fascination is not enough. At that time the Maudsley hospital housed four of the pioneers of autism research: child psychiatrist Michael Rutter, epidemiologist Lorna Wing, and psychologists Neil O'Connor and Beate Hermelin. I had read some of their papers, but did not even realize that they worked at the same place.

The papers reported ingenious experiments on perception and memory. They compared children who were then labelled mentally retarded and children then just beginning to be labelled autistic, and they found clear differences between the groups. These differences were clues to different minds. They could not be trivially explained by lack of intelligence or lack of motivation. I was completely bowled over by the fact that such elegant experiments could be done and gave such clear results. Beate Hermelin and Neil O'Connor had already worked out ways of answering questions that puzzled me deeply. For example, why do some tasks, apparently simple, seem quite impossible for autistic children? Why are they doing well on other tasks, which appear difficult for others? Why is a child who has a good memory for words unable to comprehend their meaning? I now believe that it was just these paradoxes and puzzles that cast something of a spell on me. They kept urging me to find solutions.

Forty years later, the spell is still powerful. Although there are answers to some of these questions—and we will explore them in this book—there is much more still to be discovered, and the puzzle of autism is far from being solved.

What I learned right at the beginning is that with autism nothing is what it seems at first glance. Just because a child with autism doesn't respond to your overtures, doesn't mean that the child rejects you. The reasons for not responding are much deeper. Further, just because a child can remember words and pictures does not mean that they can remember names and faces of people. One of the most startling realizations that hit me was that being autistic could be in many ways worse than being born blind or deaf. Autistic children—barring exceptions—can see and hear, often exquisitely well. But, while blind and deaf children can still receive and respond to social signals through a special sense, autistic children don't have this sense.

It is hard to imagine what it is like *not* to have a social sense, *not* to be tuned in to other people, their actions, reactions, and the signals they give out to you and each other. As it is, autistic children are not tuned into these things. However, they do have mental capacities that help them to learn about these signals. But they learn in a different way. Sadly, the knowledge they acquire is not the same as the ordinary 'tuned in' knowledge that we all take for granted. A colour-blind person can acquire knowledge of colours and name them correctly, but their experience of colours will remain different. So it is with autism and the experience of social communication.

Why does learning in autism proceed along a different route? Because autism starts so early in life, many of the social routes to learning about the world are blocked. Normally developing children can easily follow the path that has been carved out by evolution and culture. But autistic children have to find their own special routes on the byways. This makes them very different from each other as well as different from children who do not have autism.

The autism spectrum

When I first saw autistic children I was only dimly aware that autism comes in degrees, from mild to severe. Actually, all the cases I saw were severe. When I see autistic children now, I am still surprised at how many cases are high functioning and how many cases have only mild and moderate degrees of autism. To see a child with classic autism has become the exception. But I am reassured that such cases are still there, and that they have the same features as they did forty years ago. However, autism is no longer a narrow category but has widened enormously to embrace a whole range of autistic conditions. It has now become generally accepted to talk about an autism spectrum.

What is meant by this spectrum? Actually, it hides a vast array of 'autisms'. All the autisms originate from before birth, and all affect the developing brain. However, their effect on the developing mind can be very different. Consequently, there is a vastly different range of behaviours. Sometimes a family can be justly proud of their child, who is interestingly different, and possibly gifted in some special way. Sometimes a family will be destroyed because their child will be so difficult to manage that they simply cannot cope. Of course there are many shades in between, and most cases come with a mixture of rewarding and fascinating as well as aggravating and challenging features.

Every individual is unique in a multitude of ways, but they also resemble each other in some fundamental preferences and characteristics. What binds them all together, the mild and severe forms of the spectrum? At the core, there is always a characteristic inability to engage in ordinary reciprocal social interaction. There is also a characteristic rigidity of behaviour, with a multitude of consequences. That is why no one has yet given up the idea that there is a common pattern behind the kaleidoscope of individual behaviours. I will therefore frequently use the familiar terms autism and autistic, as a reminder that there is central idea behind the spectrum.

Three cases

Now we shall look at three cases closely based on real cases from different parts of the autism spectrum. David has classic autism. Gary has an autism spectrum disorder (ASD) with a diffuse and atypical picture, but such complex cases are actually quite common. Edward has classic Asperger syndrome.

David

David was 3 when he was diagnosed as autistic. At that time he hardly looked at people, was not talking, and seemed lost in his own world. He loved to bounce on a trampoline for hours and was extremely adept at doing jigsaw puzzles. At 10 years of age David had developed well physically, but emotionally remained very immature. He had a beautiful face with delicate features. Family life has always had to fit around David, not the other way round. He was and still is extremely stubborn in his likes and dislikes. At one stage he only ate yoghurt and refused all other kinds of food. More often than not his mother has to give in to his urgent and repeated demands, which easily escalate into tantrums.

David learned to talk when he was 5. He now goes to a special school for autistic children, where he is happy. He has a daily routine, which he never varies. It is hard to tell how intelligent David is. Some things he learns with great skill and speed. For example, he learned to read all by himself. He now reads fluently, but he doesn't understand what he reads. He also loves to do sums. However, he has been extremely slow to learn other skills, for example, eating at the family table, or getting dressed. David has an excellent memory. He imitates what he hears very precisely and has a beautiful singing voice. He also has perfect pitch.

David is now 12 years old. He still does not spontaneously play with other children. He has obvious difficulties in communicating with other people who don't know him well. With those who do know him, he communicates entirely on his own terms. He makes no concessions to their wishes or interests and cannot take onboard another person's point of view. In this way David is indifferent to the social world and continues to live in a world of his own.

Gary

When Gary was at primary school an experienced teacher observed that he had unusual problems in communicating with other children and could not manage to work in a group in class. Gary's parents accepted these problems as part of his personality. He seemed to be a very obstinate child, and happy to play computer games for hours. Referred to an educational psychologist by the school when problems with Gary seemed only to get worse, he was eventually seen at a clinic at age 12. The psychologist explained that Gary had a Pervasive Developmental Disorder, a category that includes autism, Asperger syndrome, and a few other rare conditions. Actually Gary was diagnosed as having PDD-NOS, Pervasive Developmental Disorder—Not Otherwise Specified. This is a category for cases that have autistic features, but not all features are necessarily present. The psychologist also mentioned Asperger syndrome when she talked to Gary's parents. They immediately favoured this label as it helped them to explain Gary's problems to other people.

The psychological assessments showed that Gary also had attention deficit disorder, and dyspraxia, as evident in his clumsiness on motor tasks. His main problems, however, were poor communication skills and an inability to understand other people. Gary was placed in a succession of different schools. In each case he was said to be difficult and disruptive. He bitterly complained about being bullied. Sadly, he was. However, Gary's classmates made some efforts to understand him. But they failed because Gary could not tell the difference between being teased or criticized.

Gary is now in his twenties and lives at home. So far, he has shown little interest in his mother's suggestions for finding a job and still spends most of his time playing computer games. Gary often says that he would like to have a girlfriend. On one occasion he had started to follow an attractive young woman everywhere, waiting outside her house for hours, but never talking to her. Now Gary's family are watching carefully for signs of inappropriate social behaviour. At his mother's insistence, Gary has joined a social skills group for people with Asperger syndrome, and he now attends the monthly meetings without fail.

Edward

Edward was diagnosed as having Asperger syndrome at the age of 8. Although clearly very bright, his teacher felt at her wits end with him. She said that she could not teach him, and that instead he taught himself, but only what he wanted to learn. He could not make any attempts to fit in with ordinary classroom activities and he refused point blank to follow the set curriculum. Edward's family had not realized the extent of this problem. On the contrary, they had always thought of Edward as an extraordinarily gifted child. By 5 years of age he had acquired an astounding vocabulary, mainly by reading dictionaries. He was rather fearful of playing with other children, but relished the attention he got from adults. His family dotes on him and he seems to share a lot of interests and mannerisms with his father. Both are bookish people and can talk very persistently about their interests. Edward started to collect birds' eggs from about the age of 4 and has developed an intricate system for classifying them.

Edward is now 20 years old and is about to study maths at a top university. He went to a private school where the teachers were sympathetic and let him follow his own interests. At school he obtained excellent marks in all science subjects. Other subjects simply did not interest him. He proclaimed loudly that literature was a waste of time. Apart from being in the chess club, he never became part of a circle of friends. Outwardly, Edward dismisses all social events as a bore. He is fluent when he talks with his father and corresponds with ornithologists all over the world, but seems to be tongue tied when faced with people his own age. Edward sticks out in a crowd, not only by his tall and lanky appearance, but also by his mannerisms and loud high-pitched voice. However, he has started to read books of manners and body language and is hoping they will improve his social skills.

Edward is very knowledgeable about Asperger syndrome and avidly participates in Asperger discussion forums on the web. He knows that he is far more intelligent than most 'neurotypicals'. However, there are signs that Edward is often anxious and sometimes depressed, and he is being seen by a psychiatrist who will carefully monitor him in the transition period when he leaves home to go to college.

The three core features of the autism spectrum

The examples of David, Gary, and Edward show how enormously varied the core signs of autism are, at least on the surface. Therefore, a lot of clinical experience is needed to make a diagnosis. The behaviour of each individual differs according to so many factors that they are difficult to list, but they include at least age, family background, general ability, education, and the child's own temperament and personality. Nevertheless, there is common ground. These are the core features of the autism spectrum, the chief diagnostic criteria. You can find them on several helpful websites. Here we unpack their meaning using our example cases.

The first of the core features of ASD concerns **reciprocal social interaction**. It is not enough to be a loner, to behave embarrassingly, or to be clumsy in social situations. The difficulty reveals itself most acutely in peer interactions. At young ages, this means other children—not adults. Adults often make huge allowances to smooth over awkward social situations. A clear sign of failing reciprocal interaction is a lack of engagement with other children.

In the case of David, the failure in social interaction can at first glance be described as a lack of social interest, or aloofness as regards other people. However, this aloofness is actually an inability to engage with others, even to the extent that he never asked to be taught to read, but taught himself. Gary is unable to read the social signals of others. He has no idea how to get a girlfriend although he would very much like to have one. Edward can socially interact with people who appreciate his intelligence, but avoids social interaction with his peers. He tries to find out about social rules.

The second related core feature concerns **communication**. Deep down, the ability to communicate hinges on a message being acknowledged as happening. One person needs to wish to communicate, and the other needs to wish to receive the communication. Communication does not have to be spoken words, but can be gestures or facial expressions. Without the signs that accompany sending and receiving a message, there can be no true communication.

David has the most severe problems in communication. He spoke late and his use of language is extremely limited, that is, he uses it if he wants something, but not to express feelings or thoughts. Gary has more subtle difficulties. He finds it impossible to know whether people make jokes from the way they talk, and feels rebuffed when he tries to talk to others. Edward is highly articulate, but he does not enjoy ordinary chitchat. His ability to engage in a two-way conversation has improved since he has started systematically to gather information about

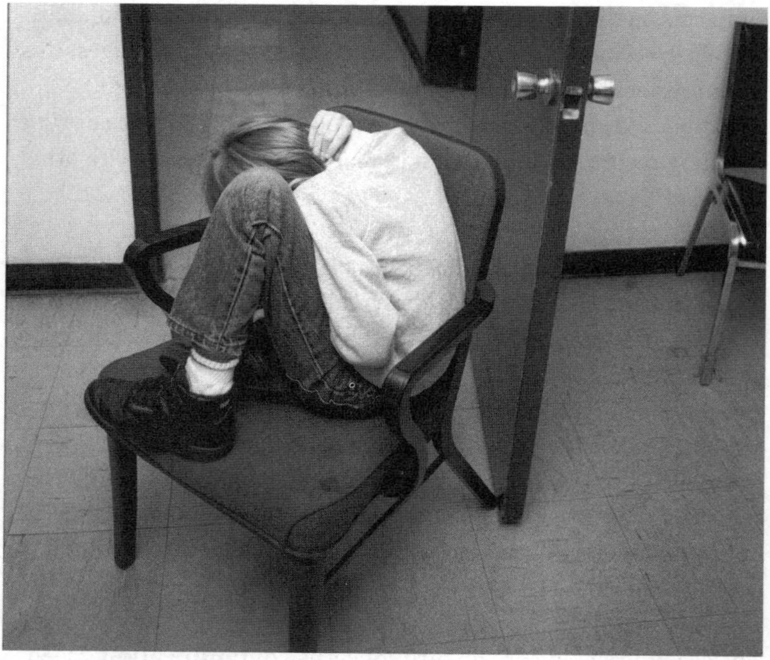

1a. Key feature 1: In a world of his own

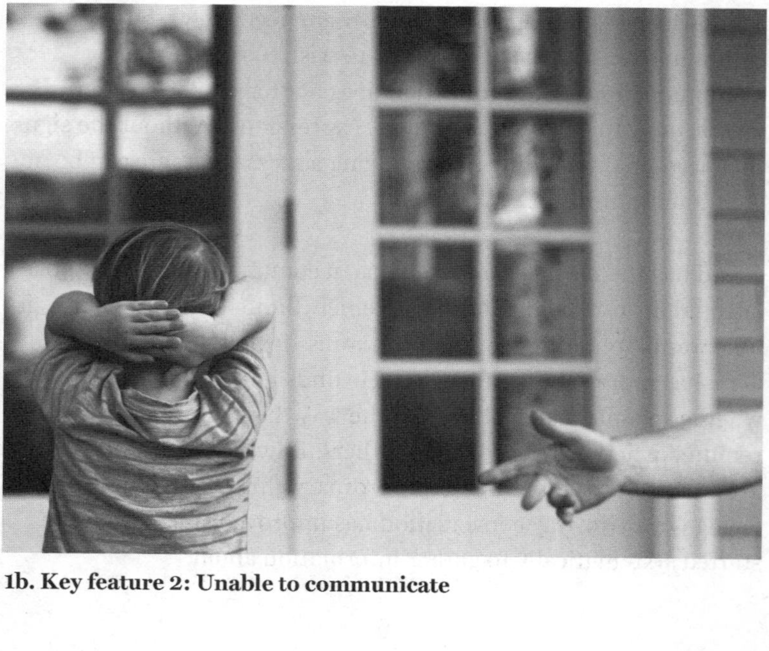

1b. Key feature 2: Unable to communicate

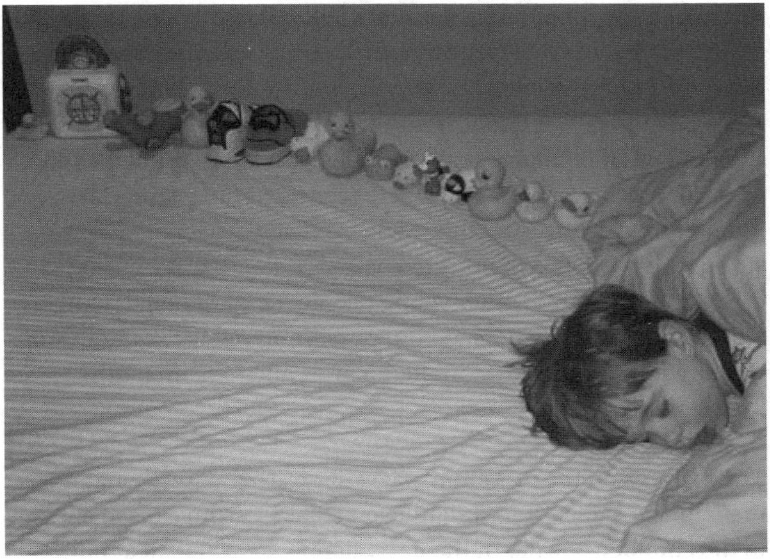

1c. Key feature 3: Restricted and repetitive. Lining up toys as seen in this charming picture has often been observed in young autistic children's play

communication, through reading books on etiquette and body language and through reading about Asperger syndrome.

The third core feature is of a different kind from the first two: it is about **repetitive activities and narrow interests**. What is *autistic* about these features, which seem not unfamiliar to many parents of young children? Lining blocks or cars up in neat little patterns may be cute just once or twice, but it becomes very sad when this is done day after day without exploring other possibilities of playing with blocks or cars. It is the extreme nature of the repetitions and the obsessive quality of the interests that are typical of autism. Another way to look at repetitive behaviour is to think of it as extreme stubbornness. In fact there is a strong resistance to change and an aversion to novelty. Doing the same thing, exactly the same thing, watching the same video, eating the same food, day after day, is the kind of excessive pattern that is found in autistic children. It is often less noticeable in autistic adults, where the behavioural repertoire has widened through learning and experience.

David's love of bouncing is an example of repetitive action and his interest in print and reading was described as obsessive. Gary did not have this feature and this made his diagnosis less straightforward. His interest in computer games was not really different from that of other young people. Edward had a number of different intensely pursued interests in succession. At one point he abandoned his interest in dictionaries and took up maths instead.

The pictures on the preceding pages show examples of what it is that clinicians focus on as significant signs or symptoms of autism in the childhood years. In the next chapter we will look at how some of the behavioural signs change with age.

Everyone agrees that autism is a developmental disorder. Development means change, and in autism it usually means improvement, an increasing ability to cope with the frightening aspects of a world that is not shared and therefore unpredictable. The repetitive and obsessive features often also fade to have a less severe impact on life. These improvements can all be expected when there is good education and support for the growing child and his or her family.

When does autism start?

This is a long and complicated story, as yet unreadable to us. Autism has its origin well before birth. At some point, a tiny fault occurs. This fault is somewhere in the genetic programme that results in a human being, with its enormously complex central nervous system. This fault is so subtle that for the most part the programme runs off smoothly, and a baby is born who looks perfectly healthy. Only from about the second year of life do the consequences of the tiny fault emerge with rather major and sometimes devastating effects.

Why only then? Perhaps, this point in time is critical for the foundation of typically human social behaviour, more critical even than the social interest that is already there in the first year. This is worth dwelling on. The healthy newborn infant, straight from birth, shows strong signs of social interest. For instance, babies prefer to look at a face rather than at a pattern, and a real face rather than a scrambled face; they prefer direct eye contact to averted eyes. They prefer to listen to speech rather than scrambled sounds; they turn to people, smile at people, show responses to familiar adults that are different from strangers, and so on.

Babies are such powerfully social creatures for a reason. For thousands of years of evolution babies have utterly depended on other human beings for their survival. And yet, the social gifts they manifest so early are quite one-sided. They cry, they look, they smile, and they babble. All these behaviours act as powerful social signals for the mother. Crying, for example, will ensure that the baby gets food and comfort. However, it seems that there is a step change in human social development at the end of the first year of life. It goes together with a step change in general physical and mental development. The baby starts to walk and to talk. Something happens that lifts the already flourishing but perhaps mainly one-sided interaction onto a different level where interactions are truly reciprocal. And here lies the core social problem in autism.

Everyone can see that in the first year of life a baby grows in size and weight at amazing speed, but we can't see how its brain grows. Almost all the nerve cells of the brain are already there at birth; it is the connections between the nerve cells that grow so phenomenally. The system is being wired up with millions and millions of connectors (synapses) and connecting fibres. The brain's communication highways are being constructed. This construction also includes eliminating bad or unnecessary connections. As the baby turns into a toddler, there is a major reorganization of the brain, and with it is a major change in the way the child interacts with other human beings.

Given that autism has social impairments at its core, one might expect that these impairments should be obvious even in the first year of life. It is remarkable that they are not. It is generally in the second year that autistic development starts to deviate from the norm, not in the first. Autistic babies seemingly stay behind and do not make the vital step change in social interaction towards true joint interaction.

What is joint attention?

There is attention from one individual to another and there is joint attention where two individuals are deliberately and simultaneously attending to an object. This accomplishment is thought by many to be the basis of true reciprocal interaction and, however social the baby is from birth, joint attention is not shown until the end of the first year of life or even later. Lack of joint attention in a toddler is a worrying sign of autism. At the same time, it is a behaviour that is difficult to induce in children who do not show it spontaneously. What constitutes joint attention?

One individual can draw the attention of another to share interest in an object and this shared interest is in itself enjoyable. Eye gaze can direct attention, and so can pointing with a finger and showing an object. One of the earliest signs of autism is that the child shows little sign of trying to attract the attention of another person by look or gesture. Instead the child appears to be oblivious to the other person present. In fact, autistic children are not oblivious. They are of course utterly dependent on other people and rely on them to have their desires and needs fulfilled. Indeed, the child can show this dependence in a most pathetic way, for instance by crying disconsolately or by dragging a person by the hand to a place where they hope to get what they need. These apparently desperate attempts seem strange to parents, when they would be only too ready to help the child if only the child gave them a small hint. But this is exactly what the autistic child can't do. He or she cannot elicit the attention in what seems to everyone a perfectly simple and obvious way, for instance by seeking eye contact and trying to engage the adult by simple gestures.

And yet it is difficult to recognize the absence of these signs. Sometimes children who have perfectly healthy brains are slow at developing social skills. Children's temperament and social interests differ, and some are slow at learning to speak. This was the case with Mickey. As a baby he did not show a lot of social interest and sometimes he seemed oblivious when called by name. This was worrying. However, on his second birthday he gave clear signs of joint attention. When his grandmother visited, he held up his new teddy to her and laughed when she pretended to talk to the teddy.

Regression or lack of progress?

Alice reported that her son Tom had spoken very early. His first words, at the age of 10 months were 'car, plane, bike'. He was a healthy and happy baby, walking at 10 months and exploring his environment with great energy like any other toddler. He acquired at least another dozen words, but from about eighteen months Tom seemed to become more absorbed with himself, and it gradually dawned on Alice that he never spoke any more. He seemed to have lost interest in his surroundings and did not progress like other toddlers. A year later Tom was diagnosed autistic with regressive development. Alice learned that this pattern of sad decline was quite frequent, and there was nothing and nobody that could be blamed for the autism. At least 30 per cent of parents have this experience.

The question is whether there is actually a decline and a regression? Or, is it more a lack of progress towards another stage of development? Could it be that Tom was like other children at first, but then other children zoomed ahead, because they had entered a new phase of mental development? Alice thought she noticed a distinct change, and she agonized about what might have triggered this change in Tom. She could simply not accept that a perfectly normal baby, who showed plentiful signs of social interest, should suddenly start behaving like an autistic child. Something must have happened: perhaps an unnoticed brain disease, perhaps some kind of poisoning from a substance that may be harmless to others. This is almost certainly not the case for Tom. Actually, it is extremely rare that autism is caused by some external agent. However, only solid research about the actual course of development of the brain in autism will remove these inevitable worries.

The case of Patricia was quite different. She was always concerned that there was something wrong. Her daughter Sylvia was a restless and difficult baby who cried a lot and slept very little. She played intensely with her rattle and gazed at the pattern of the curtains with her big beautiful eyes. During the second year, it became abundantly clear to Patricia that other children of Sylvia's age were a long way ahead in their development. While Sylvia was physically progressing very well, mentally she seemed to stay very much as she had been as a baby. Her interests in particular toys became even more intense and it was difficult to attract her attention away from them. She never seemed to look at people. She only turned to others when she needed something that instant. She never looked at her dolls and teddies either. She turned away when other children came and invited her to play. Other children pointed to objects and pictures in books and rapidly learned their names. Sylvia did none of these things.

Patricia reported later that she had hoped that Sylvia's difficulties as a baby were somehow to do with colic or teething and would go away once she was older. The frequent crying did go away, but Sylvia continued to be a poor sleeper. Patricia was rightly alarmed when Sylvia did not show interest in other children and did not pick up language.

Alice and Patricia had very different experiences with their children. But it turned out later that the development of both Tom and Sylvia was not actually very dissimilar. Both were given help from a speech therapist and both eventually learned to talk. Their mental development improved by leaps and bounds when they attended a specialist school.

What about little Mickey? Not all children are equally sociable and they don't develop equally fast. Mickey did learn to speak quite late, but he turned out to be a very friendly but occasionally shy little boy with a lot of imagination and a dry sense of humour. Diane was able to put her worries about autism aside, when Mickey entered nursery school. She could see that he fitted in with the other children, playing in the playhouse, and taking his beloved teddy for a picnic together with his friends' teddies. When she came to fetch him he rushed to show her the pictures he had made that day.

Why did Diane have to worry for so long? And why did Patricia have to wait for a couple of years before Sylvia was diagnosed?

How early can we push the diagnosis of autism?

As long as the diagnosis of autism is based on behaviour, a definitive pronouncement can only be made with hindsight. Perhaps, once a biological test is available, the diagnosis can be made before birth, but such a test still seems far in the future. Having to rely on behavioural criteria means having to live with ambiguity. And because the range of differences *between* all children is so large, even experienced clinicians can make misjudgements when pressed for a categorical pronouncement too early.

What happens when parents seek professional help, when the social and emotional development of their child seems to deteriorate or simply not move on? In the past there has often been a long and sometimes harrowing road, but now health professionals are more knowledgeable about autistic disorders and highly aware of the need for early intervention. Ideally, an experienced clinician will interview the parents about their child's development in detail, and will also test and observe the child. Then provision can be made for a programme of special education to start right away. For this reason it is important that this diagnosis is done as early as possible.

However, there is a dilemma. Researchers asked the question: if a child is diagnosed at the age of 24 months, how certain is the diagnosis? Researchers investigated how likely it is that the diagnosis is confirmed two years later. They showed that in the majority of cases the diagnosis was indeed confirmed, but still one-third of the cases were eventually not considered autistic. The study also showed that there is almost complete certainty about the diagnosis when the child is older than 30 months.

Many people feel that despite the risk of false alarms, early diagnosis is a desirable aim. One interesting solution to the problem is to proceed in two stages. At the first stage, around the age of 18 months, there could be screening for all children. At the second stage, perhaps around 30 months, a full diagnostic assessment could be offered to those children who had raised concerns. In fact, a screening instrument has already been developed. Three signs are assessed. First, does the child show 'joint attention', such as pointing with a finger. Second, is he or she following an adult's gaze. Third, does he or she engage in simple pretend play? Most typically developing children aged 18 months can master these things. Most autistic children can't. However, a number of children who apparently show these key behaviours nevertheless later go on to have an autistic disorder. This is likely to be Asperger syndrome.

In the next chapter we will consider some of the historical reasons for how we think of autism now. We will also look at the changes in what autism looks like over the course of a child's development into adulthood.

Chapter 2
The changing face of autism

A little bit of history

A hundred years ago, autism was not heard of. The name didn't exist. Of course, the condition existed, and there is some evidence for this from centuries past. However, documents that give detailed descriptions of likely cases are very scarce. The two people who named the condition were Leo Kanner (1894–1981) and Hans Asperger (1906–80), and they did it simultaneously in the early 1940s right in the middle of the Second World War. At that time the attention of most people was elsewhere; indeed the world was in chaos. The general recovery from the war took until the late 1950s and 1960s, and at this time, a handful of parents and a handful of professionals began to recognize autism in children. This started first in Europe and the USA and spread sporadically to other parts of the world. However, it took another thirty years for the general public to have heard of autism through the media.

The history of autism remains to be told. Kanner's inspiring portrayal of the features of autism had extraordinary impact. These children were beautiful, they had talents, but they also were severely disturbed and had serious learning problems. With these puzzling features it is not surprising that a powerful myth arose. This is how it goes: some children experience a rejection so traumatic that there is no way but to withdraw from the hostile world outside. This withdrawal is so complete that nothing can reverse it, except lengthy psychotherapy. Only, psychotherapy did not produce the desired effects. Gradually some practical ideas spread and succeeded in improving the quality of life of the children as well as their families. The most beneficial and perhaps also most obvious of these ideas was special education.

In 1964, Bernard Rimland's book on autism was a breath of fresh air. It championed an approach that had already been adopted by scientists at a number of medical and psychological centres. These scientists analysed cognitive abilities of autistic children, such as speech and language, perception and memory, in detail. They found strengths as well as weaknesses, and this overturned two ideas: one, that autistic children were mentally retarded overall; the other, that they were secretly highly intelligent. Clearly, they were a bit of both, and this paradoxical pattern seems to be a hallmark of autism. In 1971 the *Journal for Autism and Childhood Schizophrenia* was first published, now known as the *Journal for Autism and Developmental Disorders*. At that time autism was still little known and believed to be very rare. Nobody guessed then that in the future there would be so much interest and so many research reports that several other specialist journals would be founded.

Not only did research efforts increase, the numbers of cases increased massively too. All this went hand in hand with the increase in the awareness of autism and the widening of the boundaries of the autism spectrum. From the 1990s Asperger syndrome became a familiar label. The prototype of Asperger syndrome is the highly intelligent individual who has social impairments as well as abstruse interests. This new prototype was soon mixed up with older stereotypes of the mad genius. An idea that took off at amazing speed was that many of us, and men in particular, have autistic features. Namely, they lack social sensitivity and have obsessive interests. The boundaries of the autistic spectrum are still in flux. Will there be a clear line to distinguish autistic disorders from variants of perfectly normal differences in personality? This is one of the questions that now need to be resolved.

At the feet of the great pioneers

To me it feels that I have experienced a large part of this history personally during my own life. I have taken on board the changes in the concept of autism and have observed the huge increase in numbers of children and adults diagnosed autistic. From being unknown and obscure, autism has become a familiar topic.

I received my first introduction to autism through Michael Rutter. He taught me and several generations of students about fundamental issues of normal and abnormal development. His thinking shaped the concept of autism and spread awareness. Rutter's contributions to autism research are extraordinarily wide and far-reaching, but two are particularly noteworthy: he established instruments for diagnostic assessment now used worldwide. He also conducted the first studies on the genetic basis of autism.

Lorna Wing was another of my mentors. As a mother of an autistic daughter she had intimate knowledge of autism. I could not hear enough about her experience and her then very revolutionary ideas about the disorder. Through her studies of a whole population of handicapped children she had realized that there are three critical impairments—the 'triad' of impairments in socialization, communication, and imagination—that hold over a whole spectrum of autistic disorders. At the same time she became aware that social impairment comes in different varieties—the aloof, the passive, and the odd. She was also one of the first researchers to write about Asperger syndrome.

The experimental work of Beate Hermelin (1919–2006) and Neil O'Connor (1918–97) was the foundation of the psychological work that I will report in this book. Their ultimate aim was to link behaviour to the brain, and therefore they adapted the methods of neuropsychology for the study of children. They established a method to study impairments in cognitive abilities, such as language, perception, and memory. One of their innovations was to 'match' a clinical group with another group by equating them in terms of their performance on one test, and then contrasting them on another test. They realized that differences are only interesting if you can relate them to expected similarities. For example, they found that autistic children who remembered jumbled up words as well as other children did worse than other children when remembering whole sentences. This proved an important clue to unlocking the enigma of their minds.

Apart from these professional mentors, I have always learned a great deal from parents of autistic children. The earliest biographical account that I read was by Clara Claiborne Park. It was a revelation. Parents are the real heroes in the history of autism. They made the difference for their children in fighting for services and in promoting research. My personal heroine is Margaret Dewey, the mother of a highly talented autistic son, with whom I have corresponded for decades. She generously told me of the difficulties as well as the triumphs in Jack's life. Her examples, questions, and criticisms continuously clarified my ideas.

The awareness of autism in the 1960s and 1970s was still very low. It was much enhanced by the presence of a small band of parents who got together in National Associations both in the USA and the UK. In London these parents also helped to set up one of the first schools specializing in education for autistic children. This school was led by a gifted teacher, Sybil Elgar. She carefully observed what each individual child was capable of learning, gave clear and simple instructions, used visual aids, and encouraged physical exercise. I often visited this school. Perhaps its outstanding feature was the calming environment and a highly structured and firm teaching style, tempered by kindness.

The children in this school were pioneers too. They resembled the cases described by Kanner and Asperger in astonishing detail. Many did not talk but had some words or phrases that were copied from the adults around them. All had rather low measured IQ, but at the same time many of them showed remarkable talents. One girl had a beautiful singing voice, one boy painted marvellous pictures, another, who was unable to speak, had an astonishing knowledge of prime numbers. All the children seemed to benefit from sports activities and all took part in musical performances. Nevertheless, it became clear that these children would need support throughout their life.

Urgent practical questions: what to do about the children?

At the time virtually nothing was known about what would happen when the autistic child grew up. Now we know that autistic children become autistic adults. They too need a firm structure and a calming environment. The development of appropriate education for children with autism and mental retardation—who often had quite challenging behaviour—was of the highest priority. Some very controversial ideas were tried out for the first time in the 1960s and have since become commonplace. They were called behaviour therapy and behaviour modification, and they were based on the scientific principles of learning theory. Simply put, desired behaviour is rewarded while undesired behaviour is ignored and the reward is withheld. If such a regime is applied systematically, the desired behaviour increases and the undesired behaviour decreases. The success of these methods in managing some appalling problems, for example self-injury through constant head banging, made them acceptable and even popular.

Ivar Lovaas founded a movement in California where his methods have been gradually developed into what is now known as ABA, or Applied Behavioural Analysis. ABA typically involves intensive one-to-one training sessions. But less intensive variants seem to be just as successful, as are variants that emphasize warm emotional contact with the child. All these variants can produce amazing changes. Behaviour can be reinforced even when it is as yet barely present. For instance, parents described to me how over the course of six weeks their little son gradually learned to speak. At first he only managed to blow softly, then more strongly to extinguish a candle. Soon he was able to make some few whispered sounds. Eventually he broke through into producing a syllable, then a word. This seemed like a miracle to them, but it is an often repeated one.

There are other approaches that are geared to compensation and coping strategies rather than to shaping and changing behaviour. In North Carolina Eric Schopler (1927–2006) created a centre for the assessment and amelioration of behavioural difficulties associated with autism and severe learning disabilities. His approach emphasizes a highly structured timetable and uses pictures in a concrete and at the same time imaginative way. It is known as TEACCH and has spread all over the world. You can see the typical visual aids, depicting a series of activities laid out in a clear timetable in almost all schools for autistic children, but also in centres for autistic adults. The child or adult knows that they can always check their own timetable to know where they are in the course of the day and what to do next. This has an enormously reassuring effect and acts as a vital scaffold to organize work and leisure. Actually, different techniques—both to change behaviour and to adapt to behaviour that can't be changed—go hand in hand.

The many faces of autism

Once upon a time it used to be assumed that autism almost always went together with learning disability, or mental retardation, both terms indicating brain pathology associated with low measured IQ. Recent studies have changed this view. Now the spectrum of autistic conditions fully embraces those who have no intellectual impairment when assessed by standard intelligence tests. At present the diagnosis of autism combined with low intellectual ability is made in about 50 per cent of cases, and in 50 per cent is combined with average or even superior levels of intellectual ability.

Autism compounded by learning difficulties

Severe intellectual impairment is due to severe brain abnormality, and this will almost certainly limit emotional and social abilities as well. This is a general effect. However, there are also specific effects of brain abnormality. In autism just such a specific effect can be seen. Here emotional and social abilities are out of line and well below the rest of cognitive abilities. The case of David illustrates this very well. However, if all abilities are low-ish, then it is almost impossible for one particular ability to stand out as lower still.

Intriguingly, not all children with general learning disability, or mental retardation, have social difficulties. In some cases, notably Williams syndrome, the social interests and abilities are way *ahead* of other abilities. You can feel that there is reciprocal communication. These children initiate social contact and try to keep you engaged. The individual with Williams syndrome, even as a young child, will gaze at others, will spontaneously engage with another person, and try and hold and direct their interest. This is also often the case with children with Down syndrome. Clearly, these disorders have their own characteristic profile of strengths and weaknesses, which is different from autism.

What are autistic children with superimposed intellectual disability like? They still are a mystery, and they present many challenges to their parents and teachers. They tend to be very delayed in speaking and may never speak at all. They often appear to be locked into repetitive behaviours, such as rocking, and into routines that are difficult to break. They are more likely to suffer from additional neurological disease, in particular epilepsy. They are also likely to be less attractive in appearance, and they may well exhibit highly unattractive behaviours. The ingenuity of parents and teachers is stretched to the utmost. Such children become adults that can remain difficult to care for. Sadly they are often neglected when people talk about autistic conditions. Most people like to think of autism in high-functioning, not low-functioning, cases. But this is the sharp end of autism. Research is desperately needed to find out what exactly is wrong in the brains of these individuals, and how to improve their lives.

The term high-functioning autism was coined to distinguish it from the previously more familiar cases of mute and withdrawn children. High-functioning children have great possibilities for compensatory learning. Their intellectual resources allow them to develop alternative means to learn social skills. They may carefully observe the social rules, but still not become integrated into the complex social world. They can do well in academic subjects as long as they are taught in ways that take into account their particular strengths and interests. However, the core features of their autism are not necessarily of a milder form. A superior level of intelligence makes a big difference to the vocational achievements that can be attained, but sadly does not make a big difference to the ability to live independently. Many able individuals struggle to cope with even simple demands of everyday life.

Classic autism

When Kanner first described autism, he portrayed a type of child who is now a minority in the autism spectrum. Yet he identified a particular constellation of the signs and symptoms that every clinician recognizes. These children are aloof. If they speak at all, they tend to use rote-learned phrases and words. They do not just show simple repetitive movements, for instance flapping hands and rocking. They show rather more elaborate rituals. They develop complex routines and repeat them faithfully. More intriguing still are their special talents, for instance an exceedingly good memory.

An integral part of this classically autistic child is that it is a child—at the time Kanner described it, virtually nothing was known about their life as adults. Such a child is an icon. It is a beautiful and remote child. The impression of high intelligence can be strong, as is the impression that a normal child is locked inside. But, alas, this is an illusion. It fades as the autistic child grows up.

The autistic child grows up

Child development holds many surprises. A child can grow out of problems. A slow developer might catch up later. But more often than not children with problems become adults with problems. Slow development spotted in childhood may often turn out to be a lifelong learning disability.

The film *Rainman*, first shown in 1989, has had an enormous impact on the general awareness of autism. The main character portrayed by Dustin Hoffman is based on a combination of real individuals with autism. Many of his features were based on Kim Peek, who has become famous as the 'human Google' because of his prodigious memory. For the first time an adult with autism was the centre of attention. Previously only professionals who specialized in children, that is, child psychiatrists, child psychologists, speech therapists, and special educators—but only a minority of all these—knew about the disorder and were able to diagnose it. Neurologists, psychiatrists, and psychologists who worked mainly with adults remained ignorant of the condition at that time. It took a while to face the frightening thought that there were many adults in institutions for the mentally ill or mentally disabled who had not been recognized as autistic.

Dustin Hoffman closely observed real-life cases of autistic adults in his methodical preparation for the movie and modelled himself on them. The autistic man he portrayed was very strange, but also lovable. He looked and acted mentally disabled, and yet had the most amazing skills. He was extremely naive and had no idea that his scheming brother, portrayed by Tom Cruise, wanted to deceive and defraud him. Yet he was able to remember all the addresses in a phone book as soon as he read them and was able to win at a card game in Las Vegas precisely through his amazing memory. Most endearing was the hero's total unselfconsciousness. He did not know how unusual his abilities were. He did not consider how awkward and difficult his rigid behaviour routines were for others, and he unquestioningly accepted the harsh treatment meted out to him by others. This was a new image of autism, one that had not been brought to the public's notice, and it instantly won sympathy.

Rainman is an ambassador of autism. But not all individuals with ASD are lovable eccentrics with amazing gifts. Far from it. Many are very difficult to live with and many have additional problems. It needs to be spelled out that only 10 per cent of individuals with ASD have a truly astounding gift. The families of the other 90 per cent are rightly annoyed when strangers expect that they have a genius in their midst. However, it also needs to be pointed out that among these 90 per cent there are many who have talents that are unusual and remarkable, even if they cannot be described as astounding.

The realistic view about growing up with an autism spectrum condition is provided in a number of biographical accounts. What do they say about the autistic teenager? In many ways he or she is unaware of what it means to be a teenager. They do not have the usual obsession with looking like everyone else in their peer group and wanting to have the same clothes and gadgets. The autistic teenager retains many features that others view as childish. Yet they have the normal sexual urges. Some gain a glimmer of

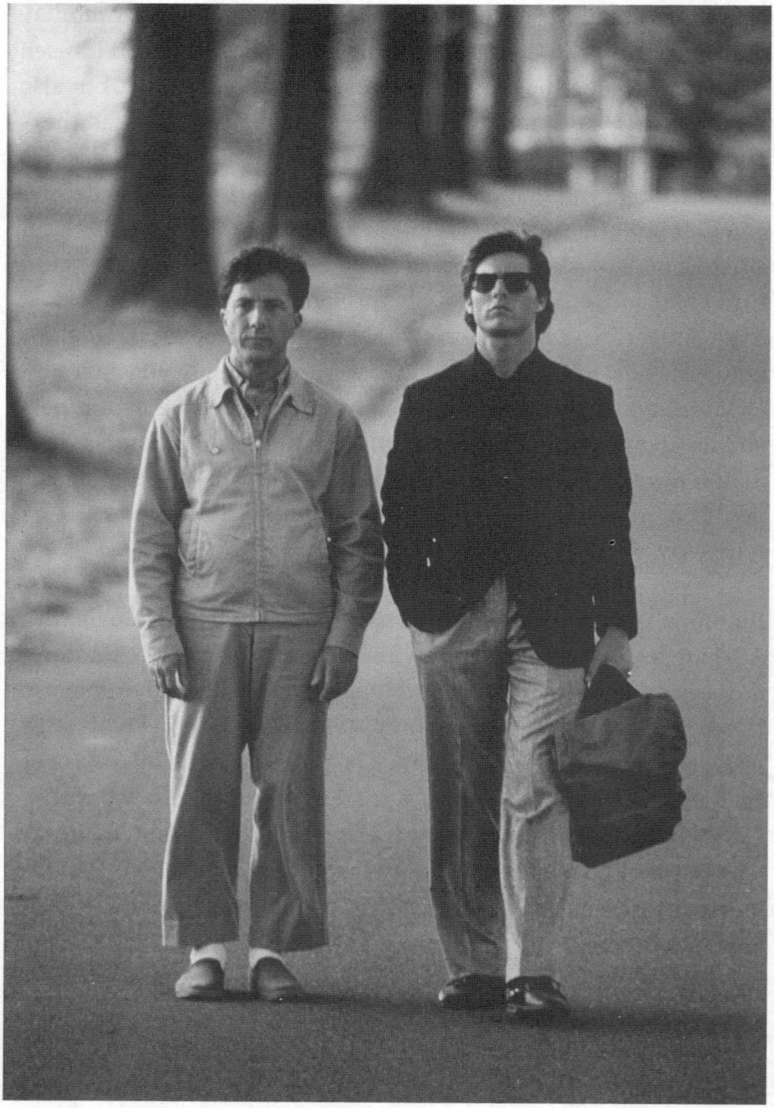

2a. Dustin Hoffman and Tom Cruise starring as two brothers in the film 'Rainman' (1989). This film raised awareness of the adult with autism and exceptional talents (savant syndrome)

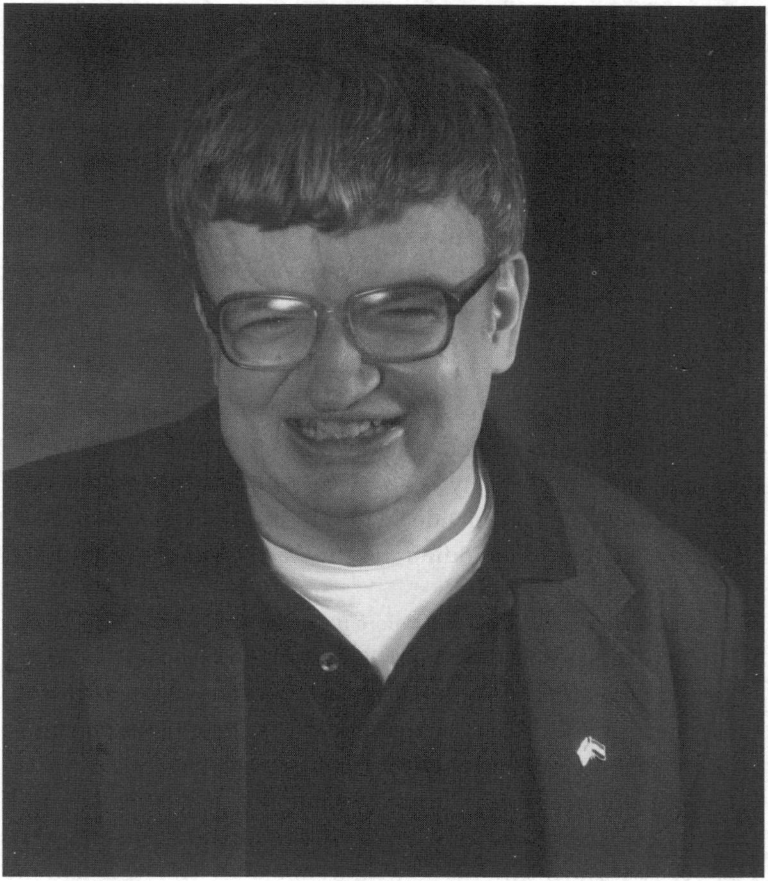

2b. Kim Peek inspired Dustin Hoffman' portrayal of 'Rainman'. Peek reads a whole book in an hour and remembers the text verbatim. He has been described as a walking Google

awareness that they are different. They stick out compared to their peer group. Perhaps they don't care about how they appear to others, and this may be why they now begin to look more handicapped. Now you notice the ungainly gait, the lack of facial expressions. Of course, in a sad way, this is helpful because it is an obvious signal to others that there is a problem.

Increased adaptation

First-hand accounts give a fascinating glimpse into the world of autism. There are an ever increasing number to be found in the catalogues of specialist publishers such as Jessica Kingsley and on websites. These accounts show that many difficulties can be conquered. Compensatory learning can lead to sometimes highly successful lives, including in some cases marriage and children. This is heartening, given that the basic problems in social insight never quite go away. According to these authors they have to be worked on continuously.

One of the most famous autistic writers is Temple Grandin, who has written many books about her own life and can look back on her experiences of over fifty years. Here is a quote from her book *Thinking in Pictures* (expanded edition Vintage Press, 2006, also published on Temple Grandin's website, easily found on Google):

> More knowledge makes me act more normal. Many people have commented to me that I act much less autistic now than I did ten years ago.... My mind works just like an Internet search engine that has been set to access only images. The more pictures I have stored in the Internet inside my brain the more templates I have of how to act in a new situation.

This self-assessment chimes in with what a man with ASD told me recently: 'There are more and more situations I just recognize and don't have to think about.'

One of the big gaps in our knowledge is that we know hardly anything about what happens to people with autism in old age. Do they have the same life span as everyone else? People with intellectual disability—whether autistic or not—usually have a shorter life span, but this could be for a large number of reasons. Sadly, one of the reasons is that they may not alert others to health problems that might be treatable. Furthermore, their repetitive behaviour may include harmful actions, for instance, drinking excessive amounts of water. On the other hand, everyone's life gets more repetitive and restricted as they get older. Many old people see their partners and friends die before them and they have to get used to being lonely, a very hard adaptation for most of us. Is it easier if you never had any friends?

Asperger syndrome

Asperger syndrome has gained such popularity that we need to give it some special attention. It can be seen as a variety of autism with similar biological causes and similar effects on the development of brain and mind, but with somewhat different behavioural manifestations. At least this is what we assume at present.

Asperger syndrome is usually considered a mild form of autism. But this may be deceptive. It may be a form of relatively pure autism where massive learning and compensation are covering up the core problems. There are good reasons for suspecting compensation and covering up. Asperger syndrome goes with high intelligence. Further, the writings of people with Asperger syndrome tell us about their difficulties and how they cope with them. These difficulties seem highly reminiscent of those of people with autism.

Perhaps the strangest fact about Asperger syndrome is that it is not usually diagnosed at all until the age of 8 or even later, sometimes only in adulthood. This is strange, because it is a developmental disorder. It does not start suddenly, but it was always there as family and sufferers almost unanimously proclaim.

Research still needs to uncover the early signs of Asperger syndrome. In contrast to autism language is not delayed, but rather it is often advanced, as in the case of Edward. Further, classic autism implies aloofness, while this is not necessarily found in Asperger syndrome. Individuals with Asperger syndrome often have a strong interest in other people. Children typically seek out adults as valued listeners to monologues, as answerers of questions, and providers of useful information.

A striking difference between autism and Asperger syndrome in childhood is that the child with Asperger syndrome displays high verbal intelligence. This is rightly a source of pride and joy to parents, but might make them overlook a lack of truly reciprocal social behaviour. Again this is illustrated in the case of Edward. As the case of Gary shows, the label is sometimes also applied to individuals with distinct social impairment who also have a mild degree of intellectual impairment. Here, Asperger syndrome is used to indicate an atypical form of autism.

What is the connection to Hans Asperger? Hans Asperger emphasized that autistic disorders appear in many different shades and varieties, including some milder varieties, and including those with high intelligence. He was one of the first people to identify and describe autism not only in children but also in adults. He labelled his cases 'autistic psychopaths' to indicate that the condition was not a disease, but part and parcel of someone's personal make-up. Asperger did not define what we today call Asperger syndrome. Nevertheless it seems fitting that the syndrome is named in his honour.

How did Asperger syndrome get its now well-established place? There are many reasons, but probably the most important was the need to widen the boundaries of the initially narrow concept of classic autism. In the 1980s a number of clinicians began to use the label Asperger syndrome. Lorna Wing in London used it to draw attention to the fact that some people with autistic disorders were highly verbal and even had some social interests. Christopher Gillberg in Gothenburg drew up diagnostic criteria to capture this particular type of individual. This allowed clinicians in other centres to identify similar cases. The criteria that are now generally used for Asperger syndrome are very similar to what in the past was considered a residual or atypical form of autism. They are in almost every respect the same as those for autism. Critically, there is no language delay, and language is often a particular cognitive strength.

Many clinicians took up the label Asperger syndrome with an eagerness that suggested that there was a real need for the category. They saw plenty of individuals who fitted the criteria. These children and adults were on the whole not so severely affected and promised hope of a better prognosis. Not surprisingly, many parents craved the diagnosis Asperger syndrome rather than autism. The popularity of the label rose inexorably.

Rightly or wrongly, Asperger syndrome has become a magnet that attracts cases. One of its attractions is that it has acquired the cachet of being linked to genius. No wonder then that a diagnosis of Asperger syndrome suggests a more interesting and possibly more tractable difficulty than autism. But this is not correct. The difficulty is just as persistent as in other autistic disorders. Nevertheless, Asperger syndrome has a special place in the popular imagination.

A vivid picture of a boy with Asperger syndrome is given in Mark Haddon's book, *The Curious Incident of the Dog in the Night-time*. This book has sold 2 million copies and has been translated into thirty-six languages. It has undoubtedly increased awareness of Asperger syndrome. Chapter 2 starts with the terse description: 'My name is Christopher John Francis Boone. I know all the countries of the world and their capital cities and every prime number up to 7,507.'

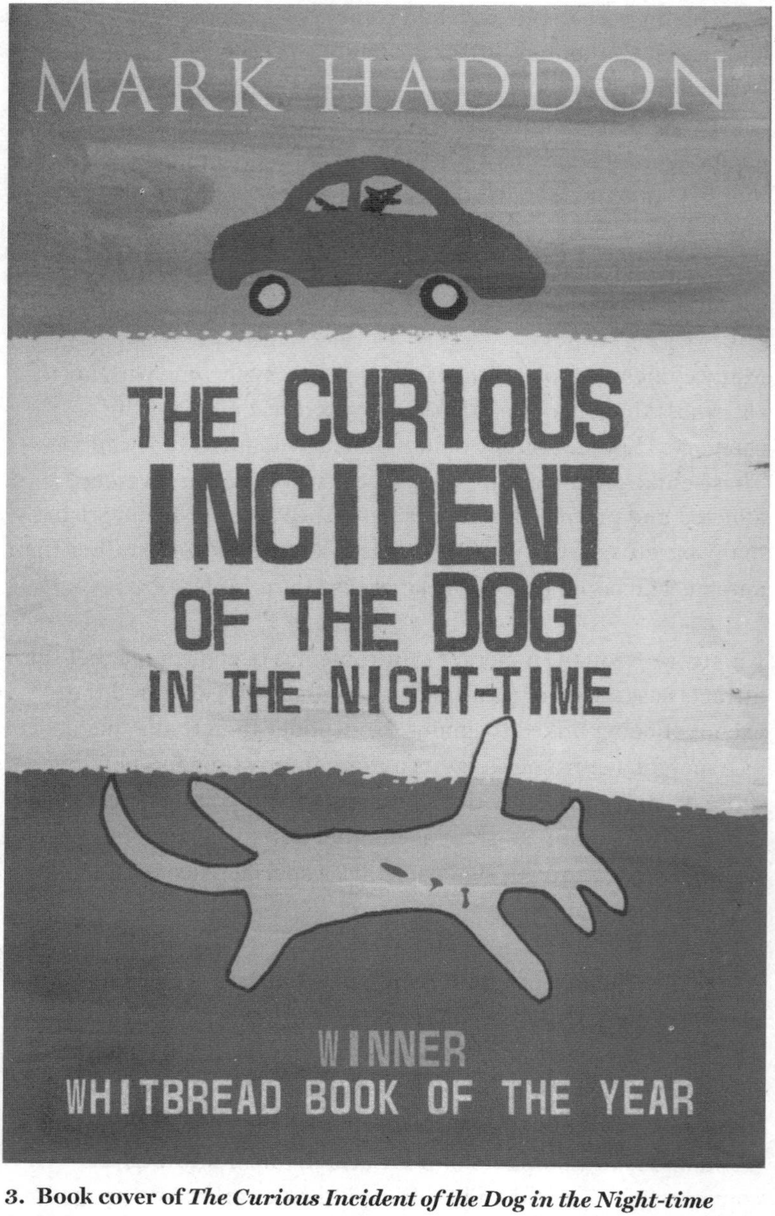

3. **Book cover of *The Curious Incident of the Dog in the Night-time***

Straightaway we are made aware of the special interests of the boy and his prodigious memory. He claims an affinity to Sherlock Holmes, because he too is super-analytical and, furthermore, he might also be on the autism spectrum.

There are many details in the story that could have been taken from real life and therefore supply telling examples of the typical features of someone who has Asperger syndrome. For example, Chris, who tells the story himself, states that he finds people confusing, that he does not tell lies, that he does not like proper novels because they are lies. He does not understand the purpose of polite language. So he can say 'All the other children at my school are stupid. Except I'm not meant to call them stupid, even though this is what they are. I'm meant to say that they have learning difficulties or that they have special needs.'

Another chapter in the history of autism

Even though it is extremely popular, the label Asperger syndrome is problematic. It is hard to know whether Asperger syndrome will eventually split off and form its own distinct category of developmental disorder. Is it indeed a form of autism and with the same genetic causes as autism? Or is it merely a personality type and not a disorder?

There are now a number of people who have diagnosed themselves as having Asperger syndrome. These individuals often call themselves Aspies, and they feel different from NTs or neurotypicals. They do not need the attention of a clinician. They are perfectly adapted in their everyday lives, occupying a niche that is just right for their special interests and skills. It is not surprising that these people argue that Asperger syndrome is not a disorder. To them it is merely a difference, and a difference to be proud of.

Some campaigners go even further and say that for the whole of the autism spectrum it is wrong to talk of brain abnormalities, wrong to focus on deficits in the mind, and wrong to highlight impairments in behaviour. Instead there should only be talk of differences in brain and mental make-up, some of which represent the autistic mind. This is a strange proposition. To someone who is familiar with classic cases and other severe cases of autism, and knows of the suffering that is associated with autism, it seems perverse. You may disagree, but then this book is not for you.

Chapter 3
A huge increase in cases

Will there be more and more people with ASD?

The one thing that frightened Diane when she was worried about baby Mickey was that she felt bombarded with reports of a huge increase in cases of autism. There was talk of an epidemic.

The stark facts as presented on the website of the Autism Society of America state that since the 1990s there has been an increase of 172 per cent of cases diagnosed as autistic. Actually, it is inevitable that there is a huge increase in recorded cases. Consider that autism was recognized only seventy years ago and became widely known only about twenty years ago. Clearly children and adults are now diagnosed with autism when they would not have been diagnosed before. Ever greater awareness of autism goes hand in hand with the discovery of more and more cases. In earlier times many of these cases would have been classified as mentally retarded.

The extent of this change was revealed in a Californian study. The decrease in mental retardation in Figure 4 corresponds very well to the increase in cases of autism. One might therefore be tempted to say that all that happened is a relabelling. However, there are also other factors at play.

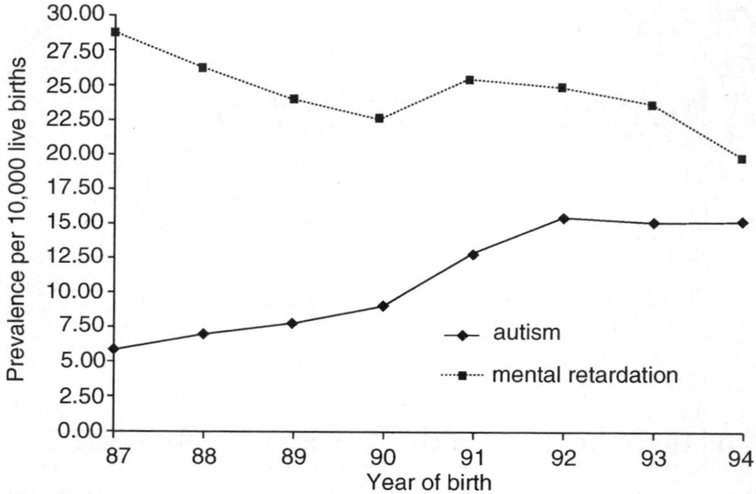

4. The increase in cases diagnosed autistic and the decrease in cases diagnosed mentally retarded in California

Croen, L.A., Grether, J.K., Hoogstrate J. and Selvin, S. (2002) The changing prevalence of autism in California. *Journal of Autism and Developmental Disorders*, 32, 207–15

One factor has to do with the widening of the diagnostic criteria to include milder cases of autism, and cases with normal and high intelligence. These cases would previously not have been diagnosed at all. If they were noticed, they would have been considered eccentrics or loners. This increase is seen in Figure 5, based on the same Californian study.

Widening the criteria

When the question was first asked how common autism is, very narrow criteria were used to identify only the most classic cases. These criteria were social aloofness, elaborate rituals, and insistence on sameness. They turned out to be too restrictive. They apply only to a small subset of children with ASD, and are observed only at a particular stage of their development, mostly between 3 and 5 years. A withdrawn child on getting older often becomes socially interested, and the reverse is also found.

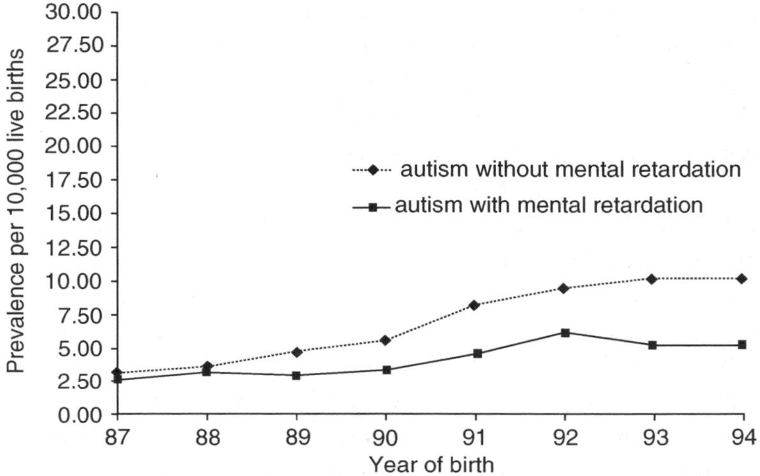

5. Cases without mental retardation increased even more than cases with retardation among those diagnosed with autism in California

Croen, L.A., Grether, J.K., Hoogstrate J. and Selvin, S. (2002) The changing prevalence of autism in California. *Journal of Autism and Developmental Disorders*, 32, 207–15

Likewise, elaborate routines and insistence on sameness can wax and wane over time.

When the behavioural changes over the course of the disorder became evident, and when the extent of individual variation was realized, the use of narrow and specific criteria was abandoned. The criteria were widened towards what is now known as the autistic spectrum. This spectrum includes very typical cases but also rather atypical ones. Young children as well as adults can now be identified, as can individuals of all levels of intelligence. Further, there are mild cases and severe cases. All this adds up to more cases.

What are the numbers now?

The most reliable information to date comes from a British study of 57,000 children aged 9 to 10 years. In this group the total prevalence of cases of autism spectrum disorder was just over 1 per cent. If you only looked at autism cases, then the estimate was 0.4 per cent, with 0.2 per cent fulfilling the narrow criteria of classic autism. Other forms of autistic disorder, including Asperger syndrome, make up around 0.7 per cent.

If we take the 1 per cent estimate seriously, then in the USA, with a population of 280 million, there are a staggering two to three million individuals who have some form of autism; in the UK, with a population of about 60 million, there are at least half a million. Assuming that about 1 per cent of the general population have an autism spectrum disorder, you are almost certain to know someone who is affected. This makes autism as common a mental disorder as schizophrenia or bipolar disorder. But unlike schizophrenia and bipolar disorder, autism is present from early childhood and persists throughout life.

If there was a 'real' increase—what could cause it?

These are scary numbers. Fifty years ago few people were aware of autism. Only the most classic form of autism was diagnosed, and everyone believed this was a very rare disorder. Now, it turns out that there are five times as many classic cases as were estimated then. Is this cause for alarm? Not necessarily. In fact, quite the opposite, if we think of the increase as an effect of increased awareness. Even classic cases had been missed previously. After all, most professionals were ignorant of childhood autism, and institutions for individuals with mental retardation housed considerable numbers of cases, who are now recognized as autistic. I certainly saw such children in special hospitals in the 1960s. Now there are numerous diagnostic centres, and there is a greater availability of services for identified children. All these factors play a part in the huge increase in cases.

Is this all there is to it? How would we know? The awareness of the condition increased gradually. So, we would expect that the

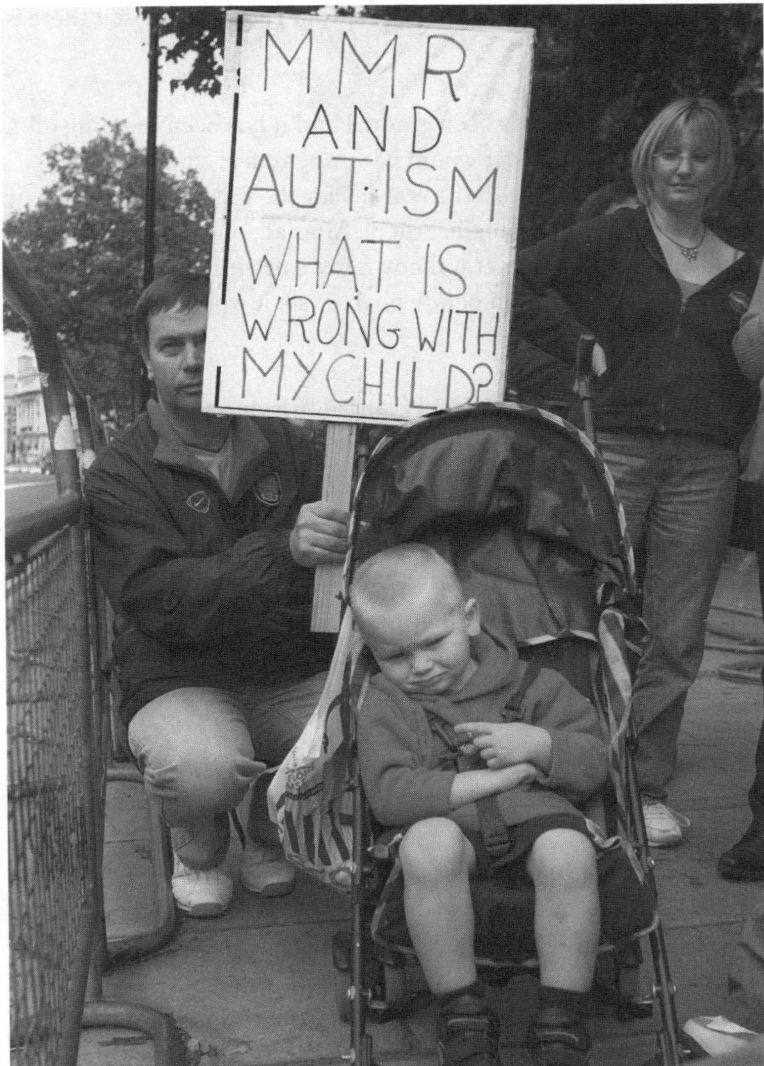

6. A demonstration of parents concerned about a link between autism and MMR

increase in cases is also gradual. We would also expect that there is a levelling off by now.

In fact the increase has been gradual and it has been levelling off recently. Nevertheless, it would be wrong to feel complacent. Parents want to know *all* the reasons for the fast and recent rise in cases of autism spectrum disorders. After all, one other reason could be a new and as yet unknown toxin or virus that is affecting brain development even before birth. If so, it would be incredibly important to find out.

It is very unlikely that autism is caused by some adverse environmental event after birth. As we will see in the next chapter the abnormalities that can be detected in the nerve cells of autistic brains date from well before birth. Nevertheless the personal experience of many parents goes against this. Remember, that many parents reported that their children seemed perfectly normal to them as babies. They had no cause for concern until their child inexplicably changed. This was sometime in the second year of life. They lost the language they already had and completely lost interest in other people.

Scare stories

What sort of unusual and possibly traumatic events happen in the second year that might cause this problem? Vaccination! Vaccination always has an aura of suspicion. By its very nature vaccination is an assault on the small and vulnerable body of a young child. In order to prevent disease, the vaccine provokes a mild form of the disease. These symptoms are temporary and soon shaken off by almost all healthy children. But there are rare cases where things can go wrong, and very wrong, where consequences might even result in brain damage. Now, if vaccinations were multiplied, would the risk be even higher? Precisely such a multiplication was introduced relatively recently. In many countries it became health policy to protect the population with a *single* vaccination against three killer diseases, measles, mumps, and rubella—MMR, the triple vaccination.

Could the triple vaccination be linked to the increase in autism? This hypothesis was clear, plausible, and definitely worth pursuing. And it was pursued vigorously in a number of studies worldwide. Almost unanimously these studies came up with a resoundingly negative answer. Study after study demonstrated that the increase in autism started long before triple vaccination was introduced. The introduction of the vaccine did not go together with a steep rise in cases. The last nail in the coffin was that the withdrawal of MMR in Japan did nothing to stop the rise of cases of ASD. In short, this vaccination is not responsible for increases in cases of autism.

Experts delved into medical records of individual cases, and found that in many there was concern about the child's development already before the vaccination. Even though the negative results were reported in the press, remaining doubts and dissenting views continued to be presented. Indeed the general concern with vaccination has still not disappeared. Are governments and big pharmaceutical corporations out to suppress the truth and deny responsibility? Does the individual ever get a hearing against a powerful corporate defence? On the other hand, do lawyers unscrupulously take advantage of suspicion to make claims for compensation? There have been precedents for both cover-ups and greed. Given previous scandals where public reassurance had been wrong, politicians feel understandably ambivalent and are torn between whether to side with scientists or parental pressure groups.

But it was not only the triple vaccination that worried people. Thimerosal, a derivative of mercury, has been used from the 1930s as an effective preservative for vaccines and for other medicines too until very recently. It has been phased out from 1999. Mercury is a heavy metal, and hazardous because the brain is susceptible to poisoning by heavy metals. It seemed possible that this could be a contributory cause of autism. This is another idea that was worth pursuing. It was taken very seriously by scientists in the USA and particularly in Japan, where in the recent past a terrible environmental disaster due to metal poisoning had occurred. However, researchers were able to rule out mercury poisoning as a cause of autism, comparing children exposed to mercury with those who were not. Furthermore, the number of autism cases continued to increase in California after Thimerosal was removed from vaccines. Nevertheless, the idea still lingers on, and many websites are devoted to this case, including those that offer treatments to remove traces of heavy metals from the body, which are themselves hazardous.

Just as in the case of the triple vaccine, some campaigners are so convinced of their claims regarding Thimerosal that they cannot change their belief. They do not see the relevance of scientific studies that refute the claims. This suggests that other as yet unknown scares could start at any time and take over the lives of campaigners.

Of course there will be more ideas about which environmental factors might contribute to autism. But these ideas need to be anchored in basic research, and basic research has not yet thrown up a credible candidate. On the other hand, blue-sky ideas about possible factors, not anchored in basic research, can waste an awful lot of time and energy.

More reasons for further increases in numbers

Here we take a brief look at the now often blurred boundaries of autistic spectrum disorders.

Diane's colleague at the lab where she worked had a little son who was 7 years old and increasingly difficult to handle. He was constantly doing things he should not do; he had tantrums almost daily; he was aggressive to other children and seemed unable to take part in group activities at school. Moira was at the end of her tether and finally went to a clinic specializing in autistic disorders. Diane was not surprised when Moira announced that Ben had an autism spectrum disorder. The diagnosis brought considerable relief to Moira. Ben was not simply a naughty child, who misbehaved all the time. Instead he just couldn't help being different. Further, she now might obtain special educational resources that she could not otherwise have claimed. But would another professional have diagnosed Ben as having conduct disorder with attention deficit disorder? Quite possibly.

What about the very bright children who are puzzling because, compared to their high intelligence, their social interaction and communication is relatively backward? There may now sometimes be pressure for a diagnosis of Asperger syndrome, when in previous times no one would have worried. In past times these children would have been treasured for their high abilities, and their social awkwardness would have been excused. In today's culture social abilities are arguably more vital to success than ever before, and therefore treasured more highly than ever before.

Perhaps today social incompetence is apparent more often because the demands on social competence are so high. Maybe our social life has become more complicated as people travel more, migrate more, and change jobs more often. If so, it would not be surprising if more children and adults fall short of high demands on social skills. This would include individuals with no particular problems of any kind, but a propensity to be loners and unconventional in their interests. Possibly such people would now be considered for diagnosis, even though they would not have been a generation ago.

We also should consider children with mental retardation of unknown causes. Here social competence is often in line with other abilities and all abilities are very limited. If looked at in detail, the poor social skills turn out not to be the same as in autism, but superficially there might be little difference. However, these children too tend to be increasingly subsumed under the autism spectrum.

I have mentioned these examples because the blurring of the boundaries brings the danger of diluting the concept of autism. This would be a pity, because research has succeeded in identifying the core social features of autism, and has provided methods to differentiate different kinds of social impairment. These are likely to have a different basis in the mind/brain. I have already touched on the characteristic impairment in autism as concerning truly reciprocal interaction.

The widening of the criteria for autistic disorder is a commonly acknowledged reason why there are so many cases today. Is this a good thing or a bad thing? The answer will depend on your point of view. Is there a limit to widening the concept of autism and the stretching of criteria? Does the spectrum really have sharp cut-off points where we can diagnose a person who is affected by autism and a person who is not?

What about the relatives of people with ASD? Are they 'on the spectrum' themselves? Sometimes quite strong and sometimes very watered down symptoms can be seen in the relatives. The observation of very mild autistic features in relatives is greater than might be expected by chance. This has given rise to the idea that there is indeed a broader phenotype of autistic disorders. This means that the genes that are responsible for this phenotype might exist in quite a large number of people, hardly any of whom are autistic themselves. Perhaps these genes predispose them to have children with ASD. This idea is plausible, but as yet speculative.

Are we all—or at least all men—a little bit autistic?

Diane can easily spot people with poor social and emotional intelligence, and most of them seem to be male. In her husband she can spot a sad lack of interest in romantic movies compared to his obsessive interest in football. He seems to spend endless hours going through websites to identify the latest technical gizmos and accessories for his camera. Does this have anything to do with the autism spectrum?

I can see the mocking humour in describing your nearest and dearest or the person next door as 'definitely on the spectrum' or 'a little bit autistic'. It conveys quite a lot of information about the person. But for me this has nothing to do with the true autism spectrum. We are usually talking of a highly educated male who can focus single-mindedly on a particular goal to the detriment of his concern for other people. This male can be an outstanding scientist or artist who doesn't seem to care what others think of him. Sometimes he is a scholar who is not particularly creative, but has the ability to acquire and retain masses of information. He will generally dislike novelty and often rigidly hold to his own opinion.

Being a 'little bit autistic' can be something of a fashion statement. It can also be a welcome excuse for people who are particularly obsessed with their own interests, and don't wish to consider another person's point of view. It can also be a great compliment. It vaguely alludes to genius. Hans Asperger himself implied that a dash of autism was part and parcel of being a creative scientist. He drew parallels between autism, scientific originality, and introversion.

Was Asperger right in claiming that the autistic personality is an extreme variant of male intelligence? In his 1944 paper, which I translated (*Autism and Asperger Syndrome* (1991), 85), he says:

> Girls are the better learners. They are more gifted for the concrete and the practical, and for tidy, methodical work. Boys, on the other hand, tend to have a gift for logical ability, abstraction, precise thinking and formulating, and for independent scientific investigation . . . In general abstraction is congenial to male thought

processes, while female thought processes draw more strongly on feelings and instincts. In the autistic person abstraction is so highly developed that the relationship to the concrete, to objects and to people has largely been lost, and as a result the instinctual aspects of adaptation are heavily reduced.

Simon Baron-Cohen in Cambridge has taken this idea further. He proposes that the outstanding fact about stereotypically male intelligence is driven by a need to have systems. He calls it *systemizing*. However, you need *empathizing* to predict the behaviour of other people and to understand their feelings.

Empathizing and systemizing

Here is a fun thing to do. You can take Baron-Cohen's AQ test on the web. You can find it easily on Google. This is a questionnaire and you have to say whether you agree with a particular statement or not. For instance, 'I prefer to do things with others rather than on my own'; 'I prefer to do things the same way over and over again'. Your answers will count towards your total empathizing and systemizing scores. You guessed it: high empathizing scores are typical of women; high systemizing scores are typical of men. Further, high empathizing scores are typical of humanities students, and high systemizing scores are typical of science students. Interestingly, scientists are over-represented among the relatives of individuals with ASD.

People with Asperger syndrome get very high scores on this questionnaire, much higher than most other people. But don't think you can diagnose yourself, your friends, and relatives! As we have seen already, the diagnostic process is a very long and difficult process, and even experienced clinicians can get it wrong sometimes.

The excess of males

Actually, in most developmental disorders more males are affected than females—for example dyslexia, attention deficit disorder, and conduct disorder. It is not clear why this is so. It is not clear whether in autism the excess of males needs special explanation over and above this general phenomenon. Nevertheless, the ratio in autism is quite extreme at the more able end of the spectrum, with 8 to 1. At other parts of the spectrum it seems to vary between 2 : 1 and 4 : 1. Taken together, the excess of males and the typically male preference for systemizing might give a clue to the origin of autism. This is what has led Simon Baron Cohen to investigate whether testosterone, the male hormone, could play a role. The jury is still out.

After all—is there a real increase?

Should Diane be worried that more and more autistic children are born now than were before? Actually, she shouldn't be. Yes there has been a huge increase, but there are good reasons for it. The increase is not a mystery and is not a sign of an epidemic. It can be explained by broadening diagnostic criteria, increased awareness, but also better identification and services for affected children. Further, if people now diagnosed with autism do not always show all the signs in their most typical form, who is to say that there are not more hidden cases that will only gradually come to light?

And yet, Diane cannot help asking whether there is not also a hidden real increase. Science cannot at present give an answer, but should be able to do so in the future. The continued careful monitoring of cases will be essential, but so will vigilance about the boundaries of the diagnostic criteria.

Chapter 4
Autism as a neurodevelopmental disorder

Why is autism a neurodevelopmental disorder?

Mental disorders that are ultimately due to genetic causes and present from early childhood are known as neurodevelopmental disorders. Diane wonders what that means. The *neuro* part of this term clearly refers to the brain. Does this mean it is a question of biology or psychology? It is both! When she sees the term neurodevelopment Diane should think mental development, because brain and mind is the same thing looked at from different points of view. The word development should remind her that we are dealing with a dynamic process. Even tiny deviations from the normal path of brain/mind development at the start can have huge consequences later on.

As Diane informs herself about autism many questions spring to her mind. If you have the genetic fault—never mind what genes are involved—would you then become autistic? Not so. This is only true for vary rare genetic disorders, but unlikely to be the case for autistic disorders. Here the gene fault gives a *predisposition* to become autistic, but what actually happens will depend on other factors. Some of these factors might make autism more likely. These are risk factors. For example, being male means there is a higher risk of autism. Others may make it less likely, for example, being female. These are protective factors.

It would be nice if we knew more about protective factors. Could these factors allow you to escape the consequences of a particular genetic predisposition? Remember Sleeping Beauty? She gets a curse from the evil fairy, meaning she will die young from a poisoned spindle, but she gets a reprieve from the good fairy, meaning that instead of dying she will fall asleep. Clearly, the good fairy does not completely cancel out the bad fairy. But it is still better than if only the bad fairy prevails. In this case, the genetic predisposition sets the programme for abnormal brain development. This starts even before birth.

The development of the brain before birth is one of the great wonders of life. All the nerve cells are born in one place and then have to migrate to their final destination. This is so complex that problems in navigation are only too likely. Other problems can occur in forming the cells in the first place. Finally, when all this is done, another danger looms. This is the process of connecting the cells to each other.

However, this danger does not stop with birth. Brain development is by no means finished at birth. Huge sweeps of brain reorganization take place from time to time during the whole course of development. Changes continue to happen so that highly efficient pathways are created to match up to the skills that are most used. These always involve making more efficient connections between cells. This is often called plasticity.

So, the brain changes all the time, just like the mind. It changes as a result of what we learn. It also changes as a result of maturation, much of which is under the control of pre-set biological processes. Evolution has already taken care of the most basic needs to survive and we don't need much learning to breathe and walk. These are automatically set priorities for the brain, and brain functions to do with thinking and complex behaviour are not top priority. Here faults can be tolerated, more or less. Sometimes, development can work around the problem and nobody knows the difference.

Sometimes, it can't, and problems become obvious. No wonder neurodevelopmental disorders are very complex and very difficult to understand.

Why look in the genes?

Diane wonders why genetic causes are so readily accepted, when there must be other possibilities. What about environmental toxins, immune responses, food allergies, viruses, or bacteria? The studies we discussed in the previous chapter showed that the environmental causes investigated to date, such as Thimerosal, are not causes of autism. Other environmental causes, such as a virus that leads to brain inflammation and subsequent brain damage, have also been studied. Indeed some cases have been described where autism resulted as a severe consequence of acute brain disease. However, these are rare causes of autism, and the symptoms that go with this form of autism tend to be rather severe with intellectual impairment going alongside.

For good reasons, the main suspect has long been a fault in the genetic code. Hans Asperger repeatedly stated that one or other of the parents of the children he saw themselves had distinct features of the disorder. However, it was only in the 1970s and 80s that proof was obtained. This proof came from twins. Michael Rutter and Susan Folstein managed to collect twenty-one pairs of twins, at least one of whom had been diagnosed as autistic. Now they could look at these twins and sort them into identical and non-identical pairs. Only the identical pairs share the identical genes, the non-identical pairs share approximately half their genes, in the same way as other siblings. Of course, both kinds of twin share a substantial part of their environment, before birth and as they grow up. If the identical twins were more often both diagnosed as autistic, then this points to a genetic rather than environmental cause. This was indeed found. In 90 per cent of the identical twin pairs, but only in 10 per cent of the non-identical pairs did both children have an autism spectrum condition. This is a remarkable result. Hardly any other mental disorder is so highly genetic.

Now it gets complicated. In almost all the pairs of identical twins, one twin is more severely affected than the other, and in at least one pair one twin was not affected by autism at all. This is not in the least surprising to geneticists. Remember, genes always interact with other factors. So, in any garden, plants from the identical seed do not show identical growth. In some cases, the position in sun or shade, the presence or absence of water, can markedly affect what the plant will look like and how well it will grow, over and above its genetic potential. In the case of human development, we just don't know what exactly plays the role of seed, sun, or water. For this reason the search for autism genes is actually a search for risk factors and protective factors. I have already likened these to the evil fairy and the good fairy in Sleeping Beauty.

In selected cases of autism mutations in small sequences on particular chromosomes have been found. Sometimes the mutations are already present in one or other of the parents. But these mutations have been identified in a small minority of cases only. So what about the rest, the vast majority? Here, multiple genes are most likely to play a role and these are hard to pinpoint.

Currently huge studies with large numbers of families are under way to hunt for the predisposing genes and to find the additional non-genetic factors that might be necessary for autism to result. But, what are these additional risk factors? It seems that all these evil fairies cast their spell early in pregnancy. Certain viral infections of the mother during pregnancy are thought be a risk factor. Rubella is a known example. An as yet unknown effect of a drug might be a risk factor. For example, thalidomide was found not only to affect the physical growth of the foetus, but also the brain in rare cases, and this resulted in autism.

As far as Diane knows, there was never a case of autism or Asperger syndrome in her or her husband's family. But she cannot be reassured, because autism really can occur seemingly out of the blue. Obviously, in other families autistic disorders can be traced down the generations through the intricate pattern of genes.

Why do several disorders often occur together?

There is another question in Diane's mind: autism can be very complex and it looks as if sometimes several disorders might be superimposed on each other in one and the same individual. This was clearly the case with her colleague's son, Ben. When Gary was diagnosed he had symptoms that could have fitted in with a number of different disorders: dyspraxia, mild learning disability, attention deficit disorder, PDD-NOS, or Asperger syndrome. Which of these labels is the most appropriate? Autism spectrum disorder tends to be the category that trumps others. This is partly because the social and communication impairments have the most serious consequences and partly because autism is most likely to attract services. But why are there such cases like Gary?

Cases who fit more than one disorder are not rare among neurodevelopmental disorders. As a basic scientist I have felt the disdain of clinicians, who know that they daily deal with cases that have more than one disorder at the same time. The term 'comorbid', meaning 'illness on top of other illness', is often used. Many professionals who care for children who have neurodevelopmental disorders feel that the diagnosis is irrelevant, but that the different needs of each individual child, whatever they are, are what actually matters. This is eminently sensible in practice. But it is not satisfactory from a scientific point of view. We need to explain why there are both pure cases and comorbid cases.

One explanation is a shrapnel effect of some initial cause, as opposed to a clean bullet. With the clean bullet, only a single brain system would be affected while the rest of the brain is left more or less intact. With the shrapnel effect more systems will be affected at once. One possible initial cause is a failure in brain development, perhaps a failure in cell migration. The failure can be limited, or it can be more general. In the more general case it would also be more severe in its effect and allow fewer means of compensation.

However, there are other explanations. One novel idea, which is still untested, is instability. Imagine that every developing organism comes with a certain degree of stability or instability. The more stable, the better the organism can withstand the dangers that inevitably occur during development. The more unstable the organism, the more likely that it will not be able to do this. Some of these dangers already lie in the formation of the genetic programme right at the beginning, and others are in the developing brain. In theory, the same dangers may have little or no effect in a stable organism, when they have marked effects in an unstable one.

This theory is testable if the inherent stability of an organism can be measured. Apparently it can be, but it has not yet been applied to autistic disorders. Inherently stable organisms can be recognized by having more symmetrical physical features and fewer physical anomalies, and these can be counted up to give a stability value to each individual. The stable individuals can adapt better when some adversity happens during their development. But of course, only up to a point. Autism may strike even a stable organism, but then this might be the only assault that this organism cannot hold out against. The result would be a 'pure' case of autism. With unstable organisms it is likely that several different adversities would affect development, one blow after the other. The result would be a combination of neurodevelopmental disorders. In the case of Gary for instance, one would expect a number of physical anomalies and fewer symmetrical features of his body, while the opposite would be predicted for Edward. I have to add that this idea is very speculative and there is no evidence as yet to say that it can apply to autism.

The brain in autism

Surely, a condition that has a profound effect on an individual's mind must leave a footprint in the brain. But where to look for this footprint? Indeed, lots of studies exist that have found abnormalities in the brain of people with autism. But what kind of abnormality? There are no holes in the head of autistic people, no tumours, no scars.

The brain consists of millions of neurons and connecting fibres. Are there abnormalities in these neurons, in their individual structure and function? Is this visible via a microscope? Should the footprint of autism also be sought in the living brain at the level of brain systems? Such systems spring into action when we perform particular actions, and think particular thoughts. Here no microscope can help, but the activity of the systems can be made visible by brain scanners. They capture images of blood flowing towards those regions that are particularly active.

Both these techniques have been used and both have yielded information. The autistic brain shows abnormalities in the detailed structure of nerve cells as well as in the structure and level of activity of systems in the living brain. But to interpret these abnormalities is not easy. In fact, we don't yet have enough information and we do not yet know how to put the information from the two sources together.

Under the microscope

Studying brain cells under a microscope, in very fine detail, is painstaking work and done rather rarely. Researchers have found that certain parts of the autistic brain have cells with an abnormal structure. For example, there is a certain type of cell which has a particularly beautiful tree-like structure, and is called the Purkinje cell. These cells are smaller and there are fewer of them in autistic brains, in particular the cerebellum. Likewise, in other parts of the brain, for instance, the limbic system, cells seem to be packed less densely. Cells in the frontal cortex, which are packed together in minicolumns, are smaller and more isolated from each other.

All these facts are still unexplained. However, an important conclusion can be drawn already. The type of abnormalities that are found in the cells themselves suggest that they started early on in foetal development. They are not 'acquired' in later development.

In the scanner

Diane volunteered to be a subject in a brain scanning experiment. She saw a picture of her own brain, looking like an X-ray photograph. Would an autistic brain look different? At first glance the brain of an individual with autism looks fine. At second glance, however, there are plenty of differences. Some regions have been found to be smaller than normal and others larger. Abnormalities have been found in white matter where all the connecting fibres are that link brain regions together. Long-range connecting fibres in particular have been found to be more sparse in autism.

The most important use of scanners is in cleverly designed experiments where it is possible to see the pattern of activity during thinking, imagining, and so on. When Diane was lying in the scanner she was shown a series of pictures. The researcher explained to her that her brain is active all the time, but when she saw nasty pictures compared to nice ones, the amygdala region of her brain burst into extra activity. This was the case even when the nasty picture was flashed up so briefly that she was not even aware of what it was.

So far only a small number of neuroimaging experiments have been done with autistic people. This is because they are difficult to do. One of the main problems is that the person in the scanner must remain completely still. They must not move their head, not even by one millimetre. Also, the scanner is very noisy and dark, and the whole procedure can make people anxious. However, the main stumbling block is with the design of the experiments. Well-controlled designs are unfortunately rare.

For example, we could ask Edward and Gary to say what emotion a person in a photograph displays. This is something that they both find hard to do. But what exactly is it that they find hard in this deceptively simple task? If you think about the task, and cut it down into components, then you can separate out different requirements. For example, to what extent is memory involved, knowledge of words, visual perception? But this is only scratching the surface. Some of the experiments to date have found differences in brain activity during tasks, which people with ASD perform well, but appear to perform differently, using their brain in a different way. Most experiments report that activity in critical brain regions is reduced in autism. This is the case, for example, when the person in the scanner is shown pictures of faces.

Faint traces of brain activity can also be measured through the skull. The methods that are used to measure this activity are EEG, a technique which measures electrical signals, and MEG, a technique which measures magnetic signals. Such signals are given out by the brain all the time, but it is possible to catch the signals at the exact time when a particular event is perceived. So, one can track in real time how the event is processed in the brain. One can compare the signals between one event and another but only by averaging hundreds of trials because the signal is so weak. To do this, researchers may present the same tone through earphones over and over again, but suddenly they present a different tone. The tiny amount of electrical or magnetic activity that occurs at this surprise is an indicator of how sensitive the brain is to differences in these sounds. EEG and MEG techniques have the great advantage that they can be used fairly easily even with young or impaired children. Abnormal responses in autistic children, for example, when looking at faces, have been found.

We do not yet know the significance of any of these findings, what exactly they tell us about anatomical structure or physiological function. Once we can combine the information from the different techniques to study the brain, we will we know where to look for the footprint of autism. This will take time.

There is no doubt that the autistic brain shows abnormal function in different brain regions, but one has to worry about the inconsistency of the results to date. Researchers currently favour the idea that the source of the abnormalities is in the brain's connectivity. One of the most important features of the brain is the massive amount of connections between different regions. The brain has to do a phenomenal amount of work to integrate information that comes from different systems of the brain. It may well be that the abnormality of brain function in autism means that this work is done less efficiently (Figure 7).

Bigger brains

Only recently has it been proposed that young children with autism may have larger heads than other children. Leo Kanner had noticed this, but this observation had long been ignored. Actually, head size at birth in children with autism is no different from other children. The difference arises later, after the first year of life. Then again, at later ages, measurements to date indicate that head size might decrease again. What does this all mean?

Head size, and presumably brain size is not fixed. It changes during one's lifetime. There are indications that in early childhood brain size increases much more rapidly in autism than in typically developing children. During this phase the difference between the

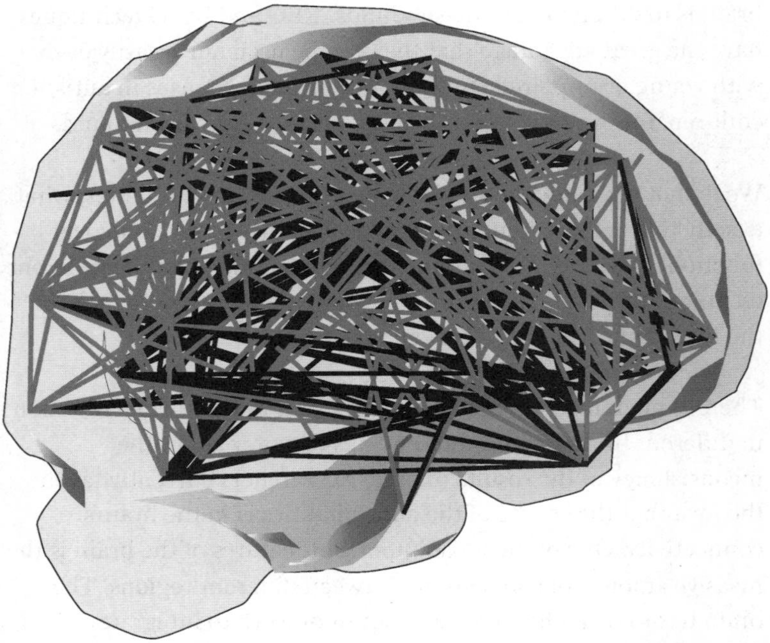

7. There are multitudes of connections between brain regions. It is possible that the brain is connected less well in autism. There could be fewer connections, or misconnections

groups is very large. However, the brain of typically developing children also increases and catches up eventually.

At this point the definitive study following different individuals over time has yet to be done. But we can assume that the young brain waxes and wanes during development. Perhaps in autism there is more waxing than waning, at least during early childhood. What could be behind this bulge in brain size?

Pruning overgrowth in the developing brain

Diane is reminded of her garden, where shrubs proliferate and have to be pruned to be kept from choking themselves. It makes sense that the brain too has phases of overgrowth and pruning. If the number of nerve cells is more or less fixed at birth, then it is

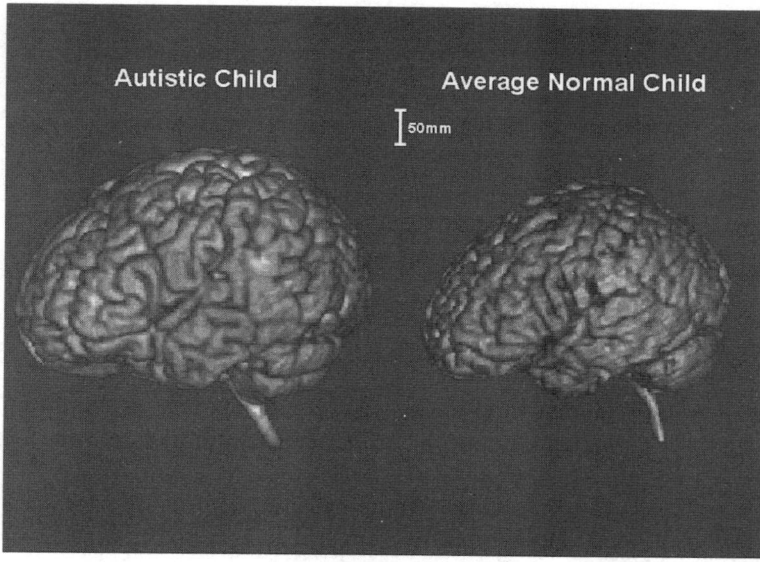

8. Example of a very large brain as shown by some children with autism. Many children with autism have small head size at birth, but show an excessively large increase in head size after the first year of life. From late childhood onwards decreases in headsize have been reported

presumably the connections between nerve cells that get pruned. These connections are quite like plants, and particularly roots of plants, with many branches (called dendrites) that spread out to make connections with other branches from other nerve cells. At the point of contact between these branches, there are most intricate devices, called synapses. These are miniature factories that regulate what goes in and out. This has all been studied in the lab of neurobiologists who can look at just a few brain cells under the microscope. Often these cells come from mice, but they work in exactly the same way in humans.

A good gardener, like Diane, often has to prune bushes, hedges, and trees in her garden. In the case of the brain the role of the gardener is partly taken by the genes that control the process, and partly by learning. Learning is a way of sorting out the necessary connections from the unnecessary ones. We can imagine that in the autistic brain one or both these 'gardeners' are negligent. Perhaps there are too many connections, which result in misconnections.

Unfortunately, no direct evidence exists that could tell us exactly what it is going on. We also need more knowledge about the normal development of the brain. There is a lot of work to do.

Some preliminary conclusions

I cannot hide the fact that there is little specific to report about the causes of autism, nor about the brain in autism. In this chapter I have therefore stuck to more general issues but couldn't resist adding one or two speculations, like instability of the developing organism, and pruning in the developing brain. You can read hundreds of scientific articles and whole books about the biological factors involved in the causation of autism and the medical conditions that accompany autism sometimes. There are also hundreds of studies using structural and functional brain imaging techniques attempting to tell you important facts about the brain in autism. However, soon there will be other papers and books, and they will all tell slightly different stories.

What conclusions can Diane draw from the work in progress? First, there is not just one cause of autism but many. Different mixes of predisposing genes might be implicated in different cases. Brain abnormalities that can be seen under the microscope suggest that they stem from a very early stage in foetal development. Larger brains in autistic children are an interesting new finding, but it is not yet known what this means.

Chapter 5
Social communication: the heart of the matter

What are the problems in social communication and why are they there?

Dare I say that the really interesting facts about autism are not about the brain and not about genes? They are about the mind. I firmly believe that even if we did know everything about the causes of autism, we would still not understand autism. We need to know what it is like to be autistic.

Why can't you fully share in the social world if you are autistic? Is there an extra social sense, beyond sound, sight, or touch, that they don't have? Children born blind or deaf can still receive and respond to social signals, but autistic children cannot do this. From now on we are going to look at insights from psychological research that lead us to the heart of autism. In this chapter we look at three big ideas that a number of scientists have put forward to clarify what autistic failure of social communication is all about.

The first big idea: reading minds

Let's go back to Mark Haddon's novel, *The Curious Incident of the Dog in the Night-time*. Christopher, the hero in the book, can solve difficult logical problems. But he does not get the social signals that are glaringly obvious to everybody else. He does not know who is lying and who is trying to help him. Why does he have these problems? This question, unlike many of our questions so far, has an answer.

...one day Julie sat down at a desk next to me and put a tube of Smarties on the desk, and she said, 'Christopher, what do you think is in here?'

And I said, 'Smarties.'

Then she took the top off the Smarties tube and turned it upside down and a little red pencil came out and she laughed and I said, 'it's not Smarties, it's a pencil.'

Then she put the little red pencil back inside the Smarties tube and put the top back on.

Then she said, 'If your Mummy came in now, and we asked her what was inside the Smarties tube, what do you think she would say?' ...

And I said, 'A pencil.'

That was because when I was little I didn't understand about other people having minds. And Julie said to Mother and Father that I would always find this very difficult. But I don't find this difficult now. Because I decided that it was a kind of puzzle, and if something is a puzzle there is always a way of solving it.

The book is only a story, but the experiment that is described here was carried out some twenty years before. That much time is needed for new theories to be tested thoroughly and for a new idea to become widely known. Scientific breakthroughs rarely happen overnight, and are rarely due to a single person. On the contrary, they usually rely on the work of many people over many years.

How do scientists study someone like Christopher? How can they find the reason for his strange problems? If you have read the book, you may remember that Christopher has to use logic to find out what his father, or anyone else, knows and believes. Only a person with autism has to do this. Most of us readers don't use logic. Instead we have an automatic indicator. Think of a SatNav that tells you where you are in relation to space. The brain has a device that tells you where you are in relation to other people. We *just know* that people or characters in a story have wishes, feelings, and beliefs and most of the time we know pretty exactly what they are; most of us are born to read minds. Christopher can't read minds.

The social part of our brain and mind normally allows us to react automatically to other people's behaviour. We don't have to think about it, but we can explain what people do by taking into account what they think and want. This has been dubbed 'mentalizing' or having a 'Theory of Mind'. In autism the mentalizing mechanism has gone wrong.

The first ever test of the big idea is illustrated in Figure 9. It goes like this: Sally has a basket, and Anne has a box. Sally has a marble and puts it inside her basket. Then she goes to play outside. While Sally is away, naughty Anne takes the marble from the basket and puts it into her own box. Now, it is time for Sally to come back. She wants to play with her marble. Where will she look for her marble? Most children by the time they are 5 years old, can answer this question with great confidence. Sally will look for her marble in the basket, because that is where she believes it is. Her belief is now false; we know where the marble really is, but Sally does not know this.

In contrast, even very clever children with autism find the Sally–Anne test very hard. They tend to say that Sally will look where the marble *really* is. They do not take into account Sally's now outdated belief. They will eventually learn what is going on,

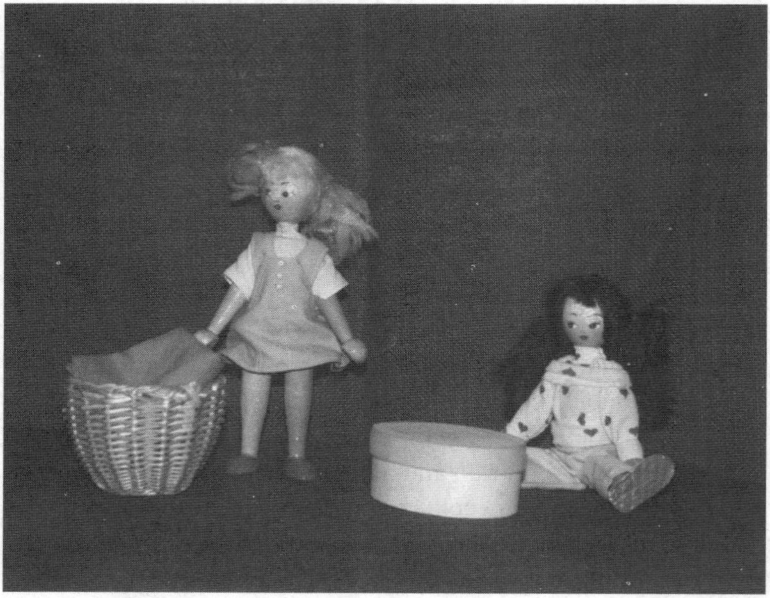

9. The Sally–Anne test

This test was used by Baron-Cohen, S., Leslie, A. and Frith, U. (1985) Does the autistic child have a "theory of mind"? *Cognition*, 21, 37–46

but it takes them much longer than normally developing children, and what they learn is something different from the easy and automatic grasp of the situation. In autism mentalizing never seems to be effortless and automatic. One extremely able person with autism said about his difficulties in social interaction, 'I sit down after an exchange to figure out intentions, beliefs, etc. I definitely need to do this "off-line", after-the-fact, not in real-time.'

So, learning does go on but it often misses the crucial point. For instance, the mother of a young man with autism said: 'I have taught him to apologize when he has hurt somebody's feelings. He always does this—except he doesn't recognize when the feelings are hurt. He is over-doing it.' But there are many cases with far less understanding. One young man was always staring at others because he believed that his thoughts would then be known to the person he was staring at.

The Sally–Anne test is an illustration of an explicit and fully conscious form of mind reading, a form that is mastered relatively late in development. Recent research on the typical development of mentalizing has succeeded in showing evidence for the ability in infants in their second year of life. This evidence is obtained from the eye gaze pattern of young children when they watch a scenario, a bit like the Sally–Anne test. For example, they gaze longer—and show surprise—when Sally looks where the marble really is, and not where she must think it is. So they obviously have a strong expectation of where Sally will look, and are curious about seeing a different outcome. Research in progress indicates that autistic children do not have this capacity for these quite unconscious forms of mind reading. Furthermore, it is doubtful if they ever acquire them. Lack of intuitive mentalizing has been nicknamed mindblindness.

Mentalizing in the brain

The big idea has led to the discovery of a previously unsuspected brain system. This brain system is dedicated to mentalizing. It was discovered with the aid of brain scanners. One challenge was to create stimuli that invite spontaneous mentalizing and contrast them with stimuli that don't do that. The extra brain activity in this comparison tells us which brain areas are involved in mentalizing. These areas are shown in Figure 11.

It turned out that simply showing people animated movies could bring out this contrast. The actors in the movies were two little triangles. In some movies they interacted with each other as in Figure 10, and in other movies, they moved randomly.

Interacting Triangles

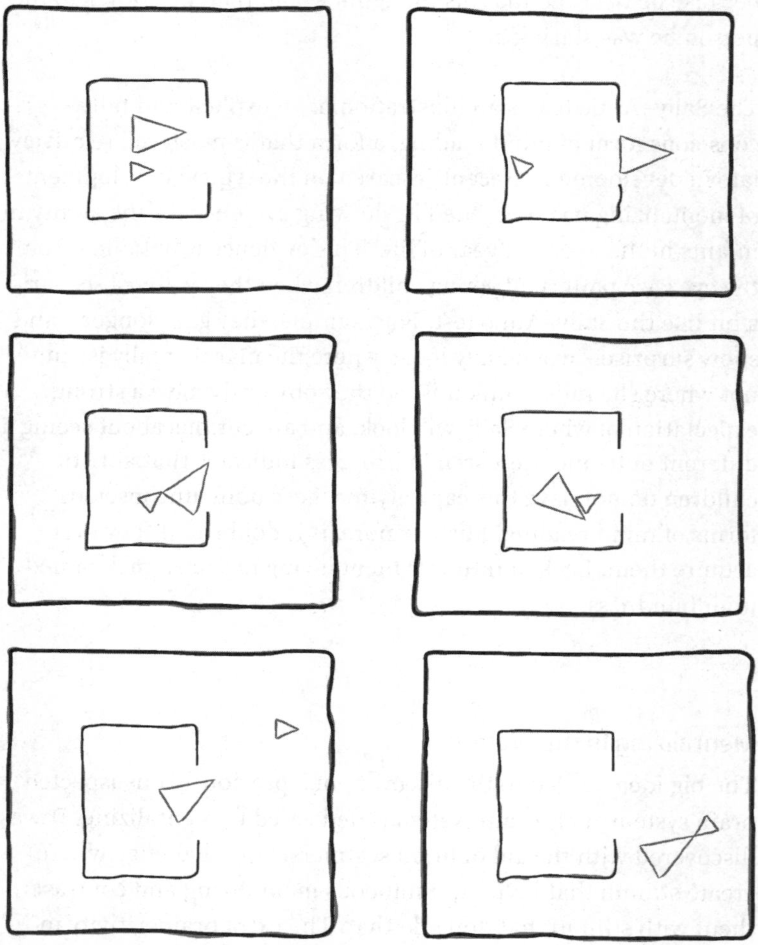

10. Movement can give the illusion that the triangles are creatures interacting with each other. The animated sequence illustrated in the stills above evokes the following interpretation: The big triangle (mother) and the little triangle (child) are in the house. The mother goes outside and gently persuades the initially reluctant child to go out as well. At last the child ventures outside, and both play happily together.

Castelli, F., Happé, F., Frith, U. & Frith, C. (2000) Movement and mind: A functional imaging study of perception and interpretation of complex intentional movement patterns. *NeuroImage*, 12, 314–25

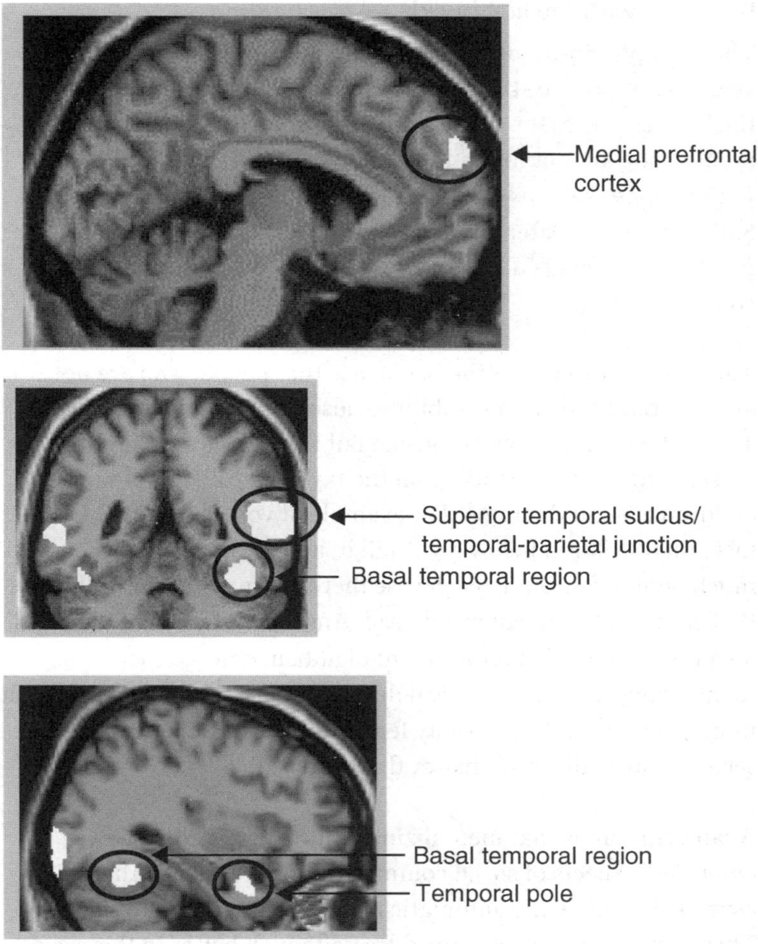

11. Regions of the brain that are active during mentalizing in the normal brain. They show reduced activation in people with autism and have weaker connectivity

Adapted from Castelli, F., Happé, F., Frith, U. & Frith, C. (2000) Movement and mind: A functional imaging study of perception and interpretation of complex intentional movement patterns. *NeuroImage*, 12, 314–25

Problems with the first big idea

The mindblindness idea has been tested vigorously over many years, but there are still loose ends that will have to be tied up in the future. One of the main criticisms is that difficulties in mentalizing are not found in all people on the autism spectrum. Let's assume that this criticism isn't just based on using the Sally–Anne test. After all, this is just one test, and to test mentalizing you need a full battery of tests with stringent controls.

The second criticism of the big idea is that people who are not autistic, but have other disabilities, also fail mentalizing tasks. This criticism is not fatal. You can fail the tasks for different reasons. After all, depending on the task, typically developing children can fail them too. For example, if you use the Sally–Anne task, then children below age 4 fail it, and so do deaf children at much older ages. But in each case there are many other indicators that show that they can mind-read. Another criticism of the big idea is that the social impairment of autism emerges before mentalizing emerges in typical development. Recent research with infants who show the capacity for intuitive mentalizing in their second year of life may answer this criticism.

A fair criticism is that mentalizing failure disregards the emotional aspects of social communication, especially those aspects that allow the automatic and intimate sharing of feelings. These emotional aspects are addressed much better in the second and third of the big ideas.

The second big idea: driven to be social

David never seemed to look at people from when he was a small child. He even seemed to avoid eye contact and turned away when he was held for a hug. He did not mould his body to that of his mother's when she tried to cuddle him. He stiffened when he was picked up. His willingness to look at familiar people increased somewhat as he got older, but still he did not relish physical contact and was happiest when on his own.

This is the second big idea: autistic individuals lack the biologically hard-wired drive to be social. Evidence for this drive is seen straight from birth. The baby prefers to look at faces rather than other objects, and seeks to listen to speech above other noises. But this is only the beginning. In the first year of life the infant is constantly engaged in interaction, primarily with the mother, but also with other people. These interactions are highly pleasurable.

One easy-to-observe example is the sharing of affect, whether smiles or frowns. Experiments have shown that infants are exquisitely sensitive to the timing of face-to-face interaction with their mother. In an experiment mother and baby could see and hear each other via a monitor. They could still interact very happily, showing beautifully synchronized movements and expressions. If the mother's picture on the monitor was frozen for a brief moment, this immediately evoked distress. The healthy young baby is a thoroughly social creature.

Proponents of the second big idea have also claimed joint attention as a sign of the hugely important drive to be interested in other people. Actually, joint attention has equally been claimed by proponents of the first big idea—as a first sign of mentalizing. Both views might be correct.

There must be a brain basis for this precociously established social drive. It is presumably necessary for the survival of young babies. This brain basis may be faulty in autism. A number of autism researchers have independently targeted regions of the brain that are known as the social brain. One particular idea is that there is a brain system underpinning our instinctive emotional responses to others, located predominately in the amygdala. A fault in this system could give rise to a conspicuous class of social and communication problems in autism. These have in common an indifference to other people, difficulties in even looking at people and, as a further consequence, no joint attention and difficulties in recognizing people.

A world of faces, bodies, and eyes

The second big idea makes us aware that we are all living in a world of people. People, with their faces, bodies, eyes, and their history, are not just always around us, but are constantly in our minds, in our memory, our dreams, and our imagination. Is it possible that this is not the case for autistic people? What a very different inner life they would have. When we meet a friend again after some years, we can effortlessly remember whether we parted amicably or had a disagreement. Imagine if you were unable to do this. You would surely think the world of people complicated and unpredictable.

Here is an extract from what an anonymous person with Asperger syndrome wrote:

> Something that most of us find difficult to remember is to whom we have said something and to whom not. Neurotypical people seem to be able to keep a mental file or record for every person they know with minute details, down to the fibs that have been said along with a mental note to keep them in mind.

One of the most important things about the world of people is faces. And in faces it is the eyes that attract our attention.

In an imaginative study scientists tracked the eye gaze of people as they watched the famous Hollywood film *Who's Afraid of Virginia Woolf* with Elizabeth Taylor, George Segal, Sandy Dennis, and Richard Burton in the starring roles. This film, made in 1966, provides a large number of scenes of intense interpersonal interaction. Hence there were plenty of opportunities to observe exactly where you look when you watch such highly meaningful interactions. In fact, most people look at the characters' eyes, often

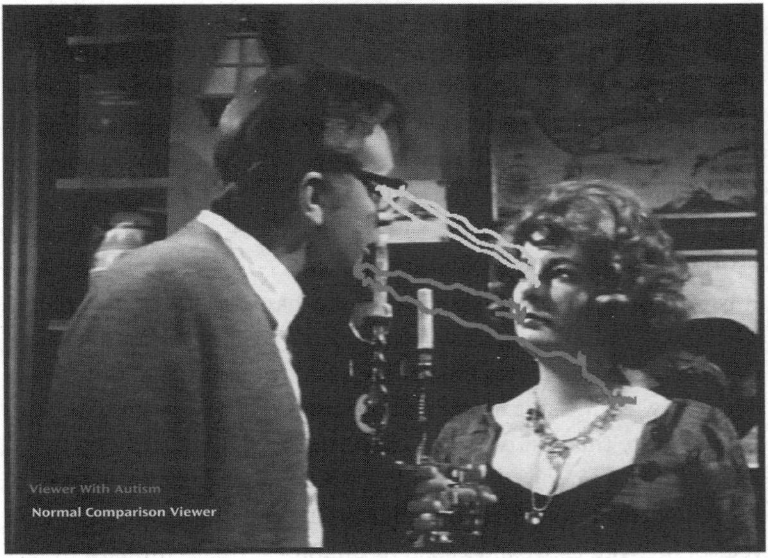

12. People were shown scenes from a film and their eye gaze was recorded. The darker lines indicate the eye gaze of individuals with ASD, the lighter lines that of ordinary individuals. The latter tended to look at the eyes for preference. People with ASD are more likely to look at the mouth

From Klin, A., Jones, W., Schultz, R., Volkmar, F., and Cohen, D. (2002) Quantifying the social phenotype in autism. *American Journal of Psychiatry*, 159, 895–908

switching from one to the other. In contrast, people with Asperger syndrome tended to look at the characters' mouths rather than their eyes. Often they looked at places in the picture that did not contain people at all.

Exciting work is being done on how autistic people respond to the eye gaze of people, when they deliberately look at objects. Normally, we expect to find an object of interest in the place where a person looks, especially if that person looks at us first, signalling the intention to communicate something. If there is no object we feel let down. This effect can clearly be seen in an increase in brain activation in a region at the side of the brain, around the superior temporal sulcus. In autism this increase does not happen. This region of the brain has come up in many neuroimaging studies of autistic brains as deviant. It is a crucial part of the social brain and also plays a part in mentalizing. Figure 10 shows where this region is located. It could well be that the underlying brain areas associated with a social drive and with mentalizing are overlapping. Future research will clarify this.

Problems with the second big idea

It is very likely that there are innate mechanisms in the normally developing brain that prefer social stimuli to any other stimuli. It is likely that these are faulty in autism. However, if autistic children were missing a social drive it should be possible to demonstrate this pretty soon after birth when this drive can normally be seen in strength and abundance. Indeed, according to this big idea, it should be possible to diagnose autism in the first year of life. Yet, as we have seen in Chapter 1, this is difficult to do. In cases of regression one of the key signs is a loss of social interest. Remarkably, parents feel strongly that in early infancy this interest was present.

The third big idea: the human mirror system

The third big idea starts from ground-breaking work with monkeys done by researchers in Parma. 'Monkey see monkey do' is a popular saying, but who would have thought that it encapsulates a basic truth about the brain? The researchers in the Parma group recorded the firing of neurons in a particular brain region. To their own surprise they discovered that there was activity in the exact same cell whether the monkey saw that action being performed by an experimenter, say grasping a peanut, or when he grasped the peanut himself. These brain cells acted as mirrors.

This was a hugely important finding since monkey and human brains are very similar. Even though it is as yet not possible to record the firing of brain cells directly in humans, we can assume that there is a mirror system in the human brain.

When we observe others performing an action our brain's mirror system is automatically active so that we are ready to perform the action ourselves. This is very useful because it allows us to understand other people's actions in a very direct way. When we perform the action, then the same neurons are active as when we observe the action in someone else.

Therefore the mirror system makes an automatic link between seeing and doing, and it is a mechanism that enables us to understand the meaning of the action that another person performs. In other words, as far as the mirror neurons are concerned they don't care whether it is us or another person who performs an action.

But this is not all. The idea of a mirror system goes well beyond action. It is exciting to think that a similar mechanism is responsible for understanding the inner intentions and even the inner feelings of other people. After all, intentions and feelings are usually accompanied by movements in the face and body. Further, does a fault in the mirror system of the brain explain lack of empathy? Empathy is often defined as a way of unconsciously copying the feelings of another person. Could a fault in this mechanism explain many of the social difficulties in autism? This is the third big idea.

There is still little evidence for the third big idea and there are both supporting and negative findings. Here are the negative findings. One prediction is that children with autism would show less good understanding of other people's goals and goal-directed actions. Also their imitation of actions should be poorer. Neither seems to hold under strict experimental conditions.

Figure 13 illustrates the success of an autistic boy in imitating precisely what the experimenter does. Her goal is to point to a particular chip on the table and even rather young children with autism can understand this automatically. They can imitate the

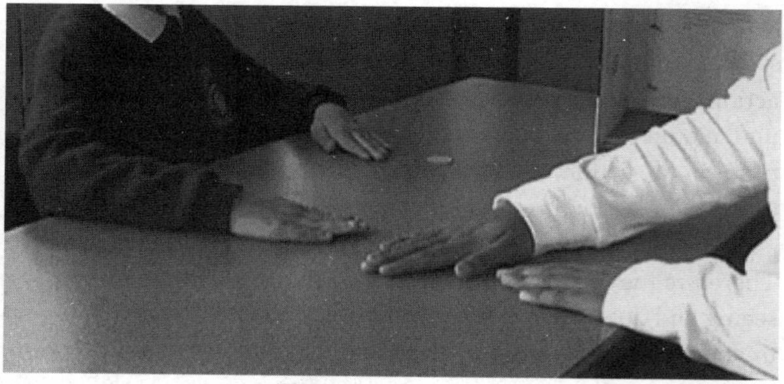

13. Imitation of hand movements. The experimenter pointed to particular chips on the table with either hand. Children were asked to copy this. Children with ASD performed exactly the same as typically developing children. They understood the goal of the experimenter and pointed to the same chip but using their most convenient hand

Based on Hamilton, A.F.d.C., Brindley, R.M., Frith, U. (2007) How valid is the mirror neuron hypothesis for autism? *Neuropsychologia*, 45, 1859–68

pointing action. Like typically developing children they pay more attention to the goal than to the hand that the experimenter used. They tend to use the hand that is nearest to the goal chip, rather than the other hand, even when the experimenter used it herself.

It is a relief to know that autistic children can understand goals, even when they have difficulty in understanding the more complex motivations of people's behaviour. However, this was an example of imitation to order, not spontaneous imitation in a typical social context. In fact, there is something amiss in autistic children's ability to imitate. There is also something amiss with their ability to inhibit imitation. This is seen, for instance, in the tendency to echo speech, a classic feature of autism. A deeper reason for abnormalities in imitation could be to do with mindblindness. Autistic children have difficulty understanding the signals that invite or prohibit imitation in particular communicative contexts.

Emotional resonance

Let's look at the positive findings. The broken mirror theory is particularly attractive when explaining why autism goes together with poor sharing of affect in social situations. People with autism apparently show less activity in the mirror system when they observe other people's facial expressions and gestures. This finding still needs to be replicated in further studies. It would help us to explain the apparent lack of emotional connectedness in autism.

One of the recurrent themes in descriptions of social impairments is the lack of emotional resonance. We all know of the warm glow of feeling in synchrony with another person's feelings. In contrast, apparent indifference to other people's feelings is surely one of the hardest things to bear when you live with an autistic person. Angela, the wife of Andrew, a man with Asperger syndrome, was extremely distressed when her father died. Andrew showed no sympathy and talked loudly and disparagingly about his father-in-law, saying it was his own fault that he had cancer, since he smoked. He never comforted Angela but seemed annoyed that she did not carry on with her usual routine. Ironically, Andrew is very aware of other people's suffering in an abstract sense. He always gives generously to a charity in Africa.

There is clearly a difference between the abstract form of empathy, which Andrew was certainly capable of, and the form of empathy for the feelings of another person as conveyed in body language, and felt as if by contagion. The mirror system seems to provide the mechanism for such a contagion.

One facial movement that is known to be very contagious is yawning. It is not even a feeling, it is a primitive reflex that does not have to be learned. Japanese researchers showed yawning faces in still pictures to children with autism and recorded their tendency to yawn. The results are shown in Figure 14. Autistic

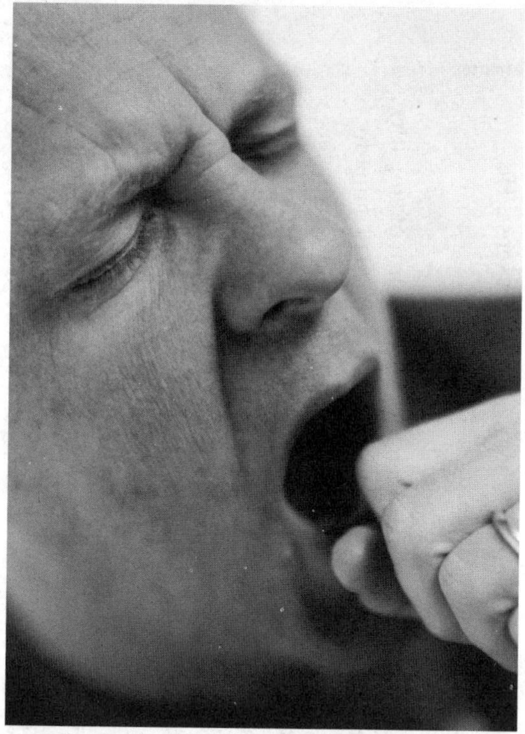

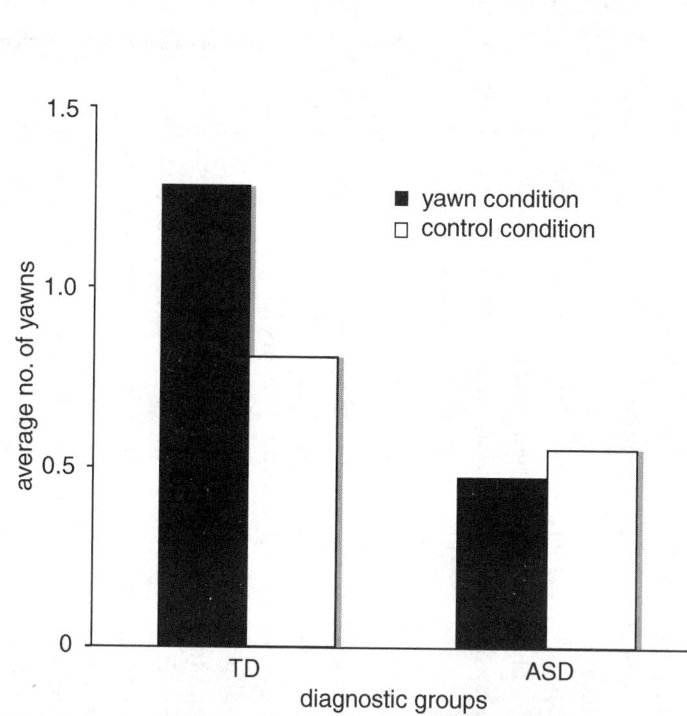

14. Left: When we see a Yawning face, we often feel like yawning ourselves. Right: Children with ASD show less contagious yawning when looking at yawning faces compared to faces simply opening their mouths than typically developing children (TD)

Adapted from Senju A., Maeda M., Kikuchi Y., Hasegawa T., Tojo and Osanai H. (2007) Absence of contagious yawning in children with autism spectrum disorder. ***Biological Letters***, 22, 706–8 children showed far less contagion than normally developing children. This finding will need to be replicated also with adults. Similar experiments are now being carried out with emotions.

Problems with the third idea

The broken mirror theory is still new. It needs to be refined to explain which social interactions go wrong in autism. Like the other big ideas, it cannot explain everything about the impoverished social life that autism entails. However, it offers an exciting possibility: it could help us to understand why in autism there is the curious lack of emotional responsiveness. It is possible that this idea will in the future define a cognitive phenotype that can be matched eventually to a genotype. It is possible to imagine a person exhibiting signs of all three cognitive phenotypes, mentalizing failure, lack of social drive, and mirror system failure. It is also possible to imagine individuals at different places on the autism spectrum, who fit just one of them.

Language and communication

Is this a separate problem in autism? Or is it part and parcel of the social impairment? If so, which of the big ideas would deal best with it?

Imagine the way we interact with a cash machine, and then imagine how we interact with another person. An autistic person would not see much difference between the two situations. This could be due to a lack of social drive, the second big idea.

The first big idea makes a different stab at the problem. Communication is truly reciprocal interaction and this is what mindblindness tries to explain. Reciprocal interaction is more than just asking and answering questions. We always probe how much our conversation partner has understood, how much he or she has been persuaded by us. We would not do this when faced with a machine.

Mindblindness has dire consequences for ordinary two-way communication. For example, people with autism don't see the point in gossip and banter. We normally love this because it allows us to do much more than exchange information. In the way we choose our words, we display our own attitudes to the world. Moreover we learn about others' attitudes towards us. They don't tell us directly, but the SatNav-like device in our brain has a sense for it. In contrast, a person with autism is geared only to the exchange of information itself. So you should not tease them, not make jokes, and not use irony. Their first inclination would be to take all remarks at face value. Note that with normally developing children there is no need to tell them not to take things too literally. They understand this quite by themselves.

It is easy to confuse talking with communicating. When David did not talk, his parents were desperate for him to speak. They felt sure the doors to communication would at last be opened when he began to use words. But, sadly, this did not happen. David now speaks, but he still does not communicate. The doors to communication do not have to wait for language to be unlocked. If they are locked, then language will not be the key. You only wish to communicate if you are aware that what is in your mind is interestingly different from what is in the mind of the other person. This fits with the first big idea, mindblindness. But the other ideas too can explain lack of communication. The second big idea suggests that communication never gets off the ground due to a lack of social motivation; the third, that this is due to a lack of mirroring of another person's feelings, intentions, and even actions. Indeed, we communicate not only by talking to each other, but also by the way we move, our face, our hands, in fact our whole body. We often give away what we feel with our body language what we try to conceal with our words.

Thus, all three big ideas have something to contribute to the explanation of the problems in communication. These are the problems that are at the heart of autism.

There is no blanket social failure

In this chapter we have looked at three different explanations for the cruel and often devastating social and communication failure in autism. But it would be a mistake to believe that people with autism have no social competence at all. In our eagerness to find reasons for the problems, we must not forget the islets of social ability.

Ronald belonged to a club for stick insect enthusiasts. Members compare notes and pictures of stick insects: there are over 1,560 species in the UK. Every street lamp has its own group of stick insects. Ronald hoped to find a girlfriend through the club. There was in fact one girl who was a member, but she was not what he wanted, not being a blonde and not being very pretty. There is nothing wrong with the ability to judge attractiveness of women in most autistic men.

Four-year-old Sebastian was almost totally self-absorbed. And yet, one day his mother observed that he brought a blanket to cover her when she was resting on a sofa. Examples of kindness that transcend the typically strong egocentrism of people with autism spectrum disorders are not common, but they exist. Likewise, examples of empathy exist, even though a lack of empathy is frequently seen as typical of autism. In fact, lack of empathy is common in people with another disorder, psychopathy. Psychopathy is an emotional disorder, where moral judgement is affected. However, unlike people with autism, psychopaths are excellent mind readers and know just how to deceive and defraud other people.

Sylvia is quite oblivious of other people—or so it seems. She does not have much social interest. She also lacks the ability to mentalize. She pays so little attention to people that it is hard to say whether she is aware of emotional expressions and whether she even remembers people's faces.

A big surprise came when she took part in an experiment that investigated knowledge of gender and race stereotypes. She had excellent knowledge these stereotypes! In fact Sylvia was not the only one who surprised us with this knowledge. The other autistic children tested also showed evidence of having the same social stereotypes as typically developing children. For example, the experimenter asked the following question about a picture of a boy and a girl. 'Here is Jack and here is Mandy. One of these children has four dolls. Which one has four dolls?' Sylvia unerringly pointed to the girl.

Besides gender stereotypes (playing with dolls, cooking, caring for others, and so on), racial stereotypes were probed also. While gender stereotypes might conceivably be absorbed by observation, the racial stereotypes could not have been based on direct experience. They are untrue! How could black be associated with being dishonest, dirty, unfriendly and white with being honest, clean, friendly? Sylvia pointed to the picture of a brown coloured person when the experimenter asked: 'Which person has stolen a wallet?' and to the pink coloured person when the experimenter asked: 'Which person has many friends?' Just the same as the other children, whether autistic or not. How did she acquire these stereotypes? Presumably by absorbing implicit cultural attitudes. This means she is not impervious to these attitudes, and this raises the possibility that unexpected types of social learning might be possible for children with autism that have not yet been exploited.

These few examples show that our social world is not completely closed to individuals with autism. What other pockets of our social world are open to autistic people? There might be more surprising answers in future research.

Chapter 6
Seeing the world differently

The savant mystery

Perhaps the most awe-inspiring fact about autism, the fact that all the fictional accounts of autism celebrate, are the savant talents. These talents can flourish even in people who have no language and are severely intellectually impaired. The term comes from *idiots savants*, literally 'the foolish wise ones', and reminds us that originally the talents were noticed in people with very low intellectual abilities and presumably very abnormal brains. Later the term 'savant' came to be used for individuals who, whatever their intellectual ability, have uncommon and unusual talents. The talents are acquired spontaneously and often discovered only accidentally. Kim Peek is able to memorize whole books by just reading them. No one had ever taught him this. I knew a boy who could look at a page of numbers of increasing size and pick out the prime numbers with lightning speed. Other astonishing examples are musical and artistic productions.

Figure 15 shows an example by a deservedly famous savant artist. Stephen Wiltshire has been filmed while drawing the cityscape of Rome, which he saw from a helicopter. You can see this film on the web. Stephen memorized everything he saw in the 45-minute ride and needed three days to draw the full panorama. He drew first not a grand outline of the map and the main features, but he

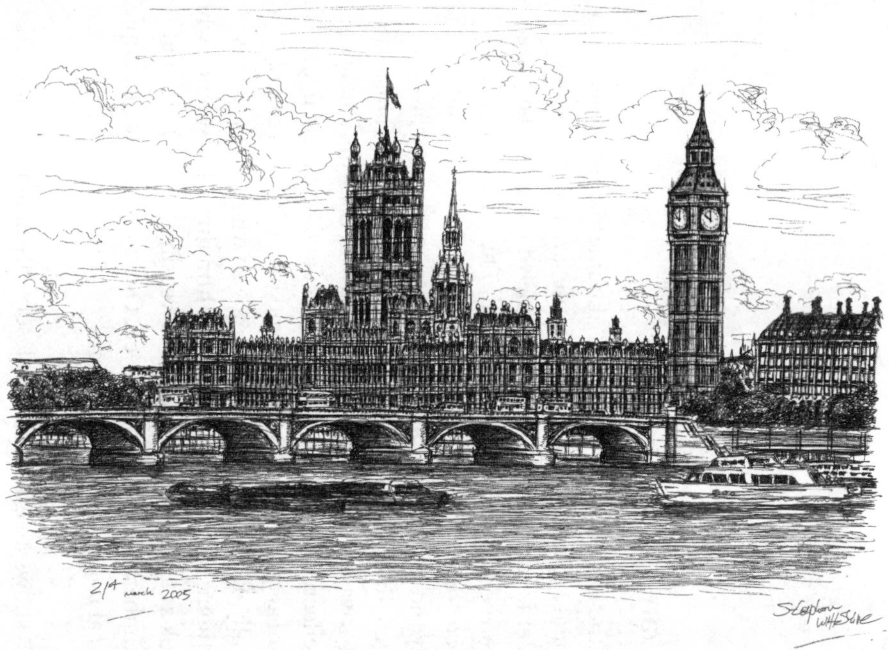

15. **Stephen Wiltshire produced this London cityscape purely from memory. Stephen's drawings are highly accurate, but they are also creative and original**

started with the detail of St Peter's basilica, in the middle of his drawing. He then proceeded to fill the surface to the right, and then the surface to the left, all in meticulous detail. In this way he created a very accurate picture, as faithfully stored in his memory. How can this extraordinary phenomenon be explained?

Unexpected strengths

Not every autistic child has outstanding talents. However, most have unexpected abilities. I recently found a message by a 46-year-old woman posted on a website for people with ASD: 'I never knew that jigsaw puzzles were supposed to be done using the picture rather than the shapes.' This chimed in with one of the earliest observations I made when studying children with autism: Some of them were able to complete a jigsaw puzzle upside down, without the aid of the picture. This led to one of the first experiments I did. I invited children to do a puzzle with a simple colour picture. Sometimes, the pieces were straight; sometimes they had jagged edges. The autistic children I tested were delighted to fit the jagged pieces together and didn't care about the picture. The non-autistic children were interested in making up the picture and were pleased when they could use the pieces with straight cut edges and did not have to fiddle with the tricky edges.

In my mind the result of this simple experiment fitted together with results of other experiments. In these experiments autistic children had to listen to words, either jumbled up in a meaningless way, or presented as a proper sentence, and then immediately recall them. Most children remembered more when they were presented as a sentence, and could manage even when the sentence was quite long. Not so autistic children. Instead, some of them remembered long random strings of words astonishingly well.

Yet other experiments showed that autistic children were incredibly good at finding hidden shapes embedded in larger meaningful pictures. Some of them love the 'Where is Wally' books and can do better than their siblings. There are plenty of results to show that autistic children perform exceedingly well on some and poorly on other tasks. Here it should be possible to find a clue to their strange intelligence, an intelligence that could appear very high and very low at the same time.

One idea was that autistic children cared for the possibly meaningless elements of a sentence or a picture, but not for the meaning of the whole sentence or the whole picture. If so, this was a completely different way of processing information. Could this processing style also lead to a different kind of intelligence? Could it explain special talents? These questions led to the theory of weak central coherence, the fourth big idea. What this theory tries to explain is illustrated in Figure 16, on the one hand, and by an example from Mark Haddon's book (p. 7), on the other. Here Christopher is clearly not as impressed or frightened by the police turning up as he should be, especially as they are going to take him to the police station. Instead, he notes some minute details about their appearance.

Then the police arrived. I like the police. They have uniforms and numbers and you know what they are meant to be doing. There was a policewoman and a policeman. The policewoman had a little hole in her tights on her left ankle and a red scratch in the middle of the hole. The policeman had a big orange leaf stuck to the bottom of his shoe which was poking out from one side.

Narrow interests and restricted behaviour

Different people with autistic disorder have written about their liking for detail and their ability to focus on detail. A focused interest in detail can appear narrow to others and narrow interests are a key feature for the diagnosis of autism spectrum disorder and particularly Asperger syndrome.

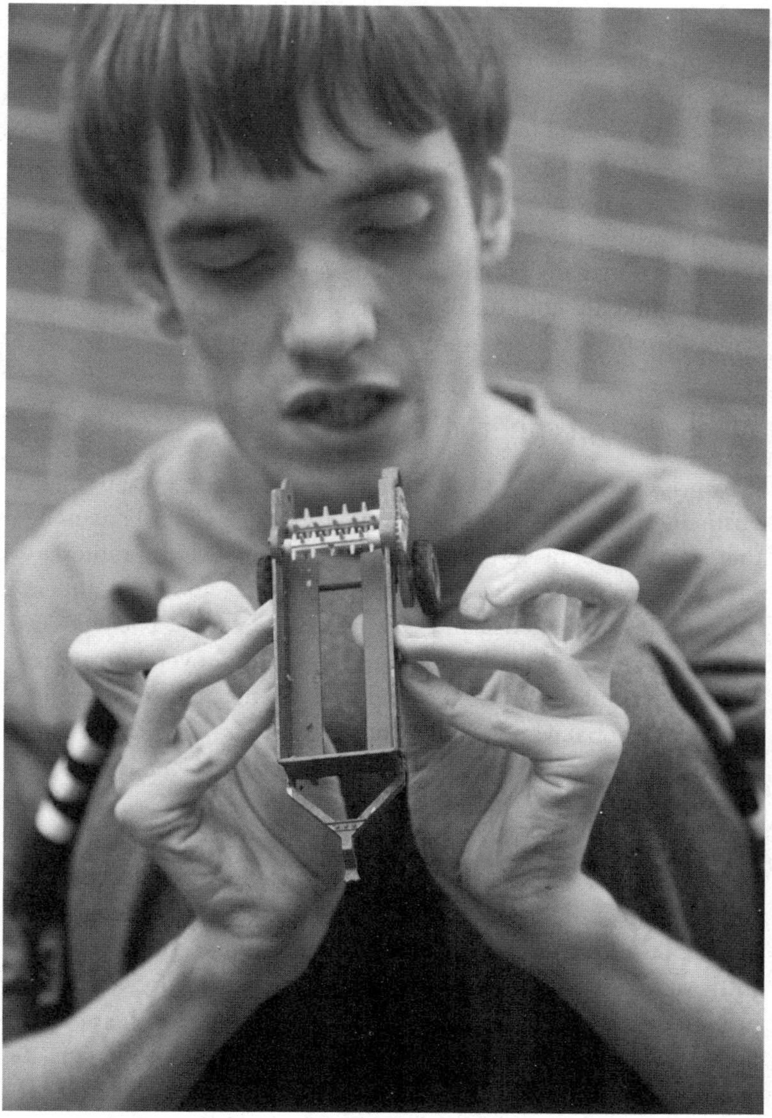

16. When the boy looks at the toy car he sees details that would normally escape us. It is as if these details have precedence over the whole object. Thus, the boy does not play with the car as a car, but is more interested in its parts, especially those that he can flick, turn, and rotate

Charles, who has Asperger syndrome, wrote in an email: 'I have unusually strong, narrow interests. This is the feature that most strongly and obviously applies to me. Between the ages of 11 and 18 I had an interest in maths that was extremely strong indeed. From 4½ to about 13 I was very interested in Rupert Bear. From about 7 to 13 I was very interested in astronomy. In the last few years I have been very interested in learning foreign languages.' Charles is unusually gifted. Characteristically, he describes interests that are not linked with each other. They have abrupt starts and stops, but apparently last a very long time.

Weak central coherence

Why is it called weak central coherence? It is a reference to the normally strong drive for meaning. With strong central coherence there is a pre-set preference towards perceiving wholes rather than parts. We perceive a drawing of an object and not a jumble of lines; we hear a sentence and not a jumble of words. The whole is often referred to as a Gestalt, a German term for overall form. It is used by psychologists to explain why we are normally geared to perceiving global wholes rather than local parts. However, it is only possible to show this preference when there is too much information and you can't do both at the same time.

Context is another way of describing the whole or Gestalt and its relationship to the parts. The context gives meaning to the parts. A single note of music may sound very loud when preceded by a very softly played part. The same note may sound very soft, when preceded by a loudly played part. The same is true for the pitch of tones. Absolute pitch is the ability to hear a tone exactly as it is, regardless of its context. Amazingly, about 30 per cent of individuals with autism, not trained in music, have this ability.

Weak central coherence (WCC) is a way of saying that context does not exert much force. The bits and pieces set inside a particular context are seen as what they are—the same—even if they look quite different in another context. With strong central coherence, the meaning of an element can be altered so much that it sometimes cannot be recognized as the same piece in another context. The illusion, shown in Figure 17, is a good example. Here the circle in the middle looks either big or small according to the context of the surrounding circles. Actually it is exactly the same size. If you see it as the same size, you would have demonstrated weak central coherence. You are less taken in by the illusion! Obviously, not being influenced by overall context can be a great strength. Sometimes, the word *weak* in WCC is misunderstood as meaning 'poor'. In fact most of the tests of WCC are geared to show good or superior performance.

Figure 17 also shows other visual tests, on which autistic individuals perform well. What they have in common is that they favour a strategy that automatically focuses on detail. This is the way Francesca Happé refers to it. She has done a great deal of theoretical and experimental work on this idea. For instance, she showed that this information-processing style is also typical of a proportion of the normal population, and around half of fathers and a third of mothers of autistic children.

Another task from Francesca Happé's lab is as follows. Complete the sentence: You can go hunting with a knife and...

If you say 'fork', you have given an example of weak central coherence, in this case an association of local elements. Knife and fork go together. At the same time you have ignored the overall meaning of the sentence. If you said something like 'catch a bear', you showed evidence of strong central coherence. Another example is: 'the sea tastes of salt and...'

Did you say 'pepper'? Again this is an example of weak central coherence. If you said something like 'fish', then you have taken the whole sentence meaning into account and this is a sign of strong central coherence.

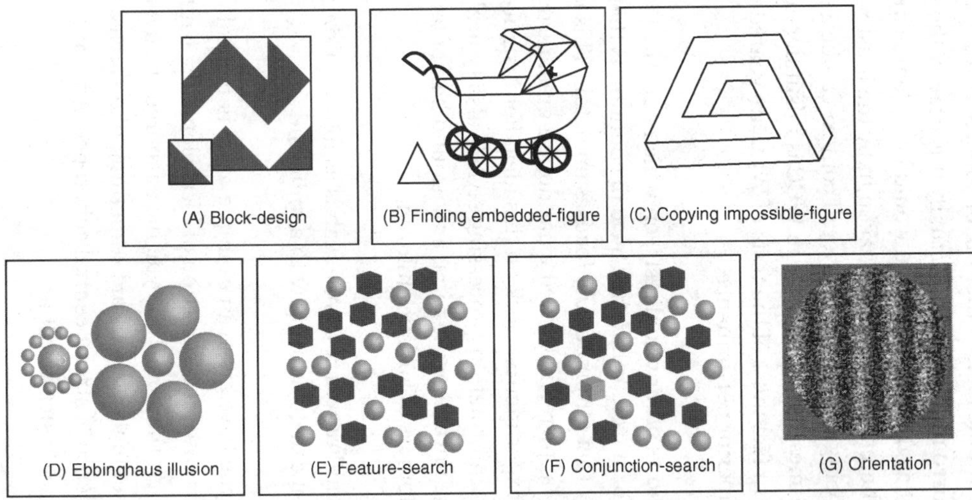

17. Tasks on which superior perfomance is often found in individuals with ASD. From Dakin, S. & Frith, U. (2005) Vagaries of visual perception in autism. *Neuron*, 48, 497–507

According to WCC, the fourth big idea, autistic people perceive the world differently. A detail-focused processing style not only applies to vision. It also applies to hearing and to language. What about other senses—touch, for example? Here an intriguing phenomenon is that many people with autism are reported to be hypersensitive to touch. Possibly, having hyper-acute touch might be a bit like having absolute pitch.

Can weak central coherence explain savant skills? Up to a point. The ability to remember materials verbatim without understanding the content is a chief example of this style of processing information. Clearly other factors must play a role as well—practice, for instance. Repeated practice, even obsessive practice, would not be a chore for an individual who has a restricted repertoire of interests and activities. The avoidance of novelty that can be seen as typical of autism also facilitates practice. When David started to be fascinated with print, he read the *Cat in the Hat* hundreds of times. He knew it by heart, but he still reread every page of it. His ability to read words far outstripped his ability to understand them.

Weak central coherence theory tries something very daring. It tries to make sense out of a number of quite disparate aspects of autistic intelligence. It tries to account both for special talents but also for certain cognitive weaknesses. Maybe because it tries to do this all at once, it does not succeed as well as the first three big ideas we looked at, which only addressed weaknesses.

It is possible that systematic studies of attention will clarify the phenomena addressed by the weak central coherence idea. Attention to details and wholes may be quite different in nature. What happens to attention when it switches from focusing on a small element to focusing on the large whole? And vice versa? Studies suggest that autistic individuals are generally more ready to zoom in on the small element, but less able to zoom out to attend to the large whole.

Problems with the idea

Researchers have tried a number of tasks that apparently show that autistic people have no difficulty with perceiving a Gestalt. Instead there is an enhancement of the facility with which details are processed. In contrast to weak central coherence, this theory is called enhanced perceptual facilitation theory. It proposes that there is a *superiority* of detail processing in its own right, not simply a result of an *inferiority* of Gestalt processing. Systemizing is another idea that emphasizes that autistic people do not just see little details but love systems. It is this love of systems that may explain savant skills such as calendar calculation.

Another criticism is that a detail-focused processing style seems to apply only to some but not all individuals with autistic disorder. As we have seen with the other big ideas, this criticism is not necessarily fatal: none of them are likely to apply to all cases of autism spectrum disorder. There are bound to be subgroups.

Trouble at the top

It is time to turn to the last of the five big ideas, the idea of a fault in the executive system of the brain. If control is absent, then you get behaviour that is out of bounds. *You get stuck* and it is hard to get out of this. Further, you are *captured by incidentals*. You act on impulse, rather than showing foresight and planning. You don't stop and think, to find a novel solution when normal routines fail. On the other hand you *lack inhibition*, and show behaviour that is not socially acceptable. Clearly, if the executive system fails then you have problems in controlling other brain systems. This idea tries to explain the many problems that people with autism have in managing the stresses of our complex everyday life. One might have thought that such problems will only be found in low-functioning cases. But no, they are pernicious in the way they blight the lives of both low- and high-functioning people.

Gary, who was desperate to have a girlfriend, was unable to stop himself from obsessively following an attractive woman. He was told it was wrong. The woman complained to the police. He was severely reprimanded and yet his family could not trust him not to do it again. They have to closely monitor his activities. Why can he not inhibit his perfectly normal impulse?

Neuropsychologists are familiar with this sort of problem from patients with damage to the frontal lobes of the brain. Patients with frontal lobe damage are very puzzling. On ordinary IQ tests they score perfectly well, but in everyday life they make poor decisions, don't make proper plans, and generally show that they are not able to use their intelligence to adapt to their circumstances.

The role of the frontal lobes of the brain is to make high-level executive decisions. These decisions are necessary whenever routine actions are not appropriate or have to be interrupted and overridden. Here are some of the typical problems in everyday life that are all to do with trouble in this high-level control system.

Getting stuck

You cannot read a better account of this problem than the one Michael Blastland has given of his son Joe. During a long phase he would only eat one particular brand of Ricotta and Spinach pasta. He refused other food, even when he was hungry. He was so desperate about this one and only food that he could sometimes not wait for it to get cooked. Blastland also tells of Joe's insistence on watching videos over and over again. The harrowing part of this story is that Joe behaved in many ways like an addict. He craved the videos. He was inconsolable when he did not get them. And yet, when he watched them, they did not make him happy. Joe's parents were at a loss as to how to deal with these cravings and the strong dislike of anything new. Fortunately, as Joe grew up, and went to a special school, these problems lessened. Joe eventually learned to eat other foods and learned to enjoy a whole variety of activities.

Captured by incidentals

'Whenever Bob was passing a house or other building and saw an open door, he would walk through it to investigate. Needless to say, this behaviour often led to unpleasant confrontations, but apparently he was surprised every time and never learnt not to do it.' This is an example of what is often called stimulus-driven behaviour. Yet, much of our everyday perfectly normal behaviour is stimulus driven. The difference from autism is that we can keep this behaviour under control. For a person with autism it is a huge effort to inhibit certain actions when they are triggered accidentally by something that has triggered them before.

Lack of inhibition

Matthew's mother told me that she had a huge battle with him every day to get rid of rubbish. Matthew would not agree to throw anything away, not even envelopes or wrapping paper, let alone newspapers and plastic bags. This sort of problem is also sometimes seen with patients where strokes have caused lesions in the middle of the front of the brain. These patients start collecting useless things after the accident that caused their lesion. This does not mean that these particular areas of the brain are the basis of collecting behaviour. Rather, they are the basis of *inhibiting* collecting behaviour, and these patients have problems in inhibition. In the brain of rats, and presumably humans as well, there are regions deep in the brain, so-called subcortical regions, which are responsible for the drive to acquire and collect. This drive is normally controlled and kept within reasonable bounds. But this requires intact frontal lobes.

Disaster zones

Ken is stressed out when he has to do his shopping. Even though he has made a list, so as not to be tempted to buy unnecessary

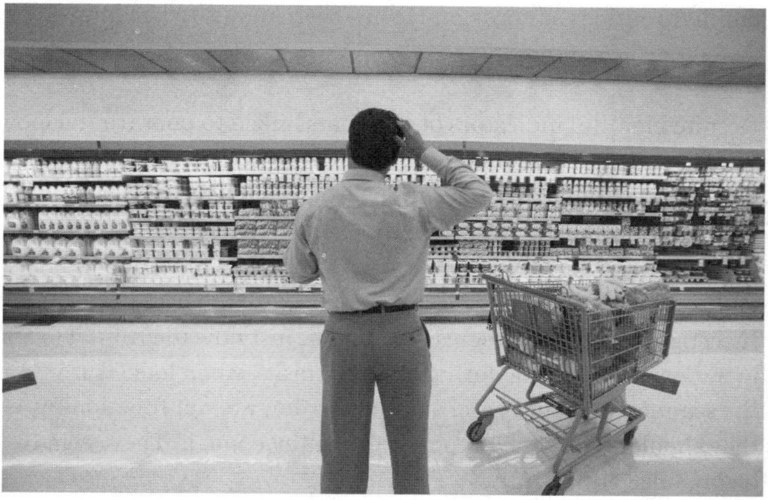

18. In a supermarket executive functions are challenged by having to plan to be within a budget; to resist impulse buying; to inhibit responses to special offers; to substitute alternatives for unavailable items. Individuals with autism find this situation very stressful, but they can follow a set routine

items, things can still go wrong. One day his brand of muesli was not on the usual shelf. Panic. Ken had no idea that it would have been perfectly alright to ask an assistant if there was some more coming in, or whether it had been put on another shelf. He had been told not to bother the assistants with questions on previous occasions. So he went home in deep frustration. This relatively mild example may give some idea how many everyday life events that demand flexibility can become major stress points. It is a peculiar lack of mental flexibility which makes their lives difficult, even in people who are otherwise very able.

Because the frontal lobes are so large and because their function is a supervisory one, the effects of damage to the frontal lobes are at once subtle and far-reaching. Impairments are found when the patients have to act spontaneously, or in a novel or unstructured situation. This is also the case for Ken. He cannot cope when his familiar routines are broken. He has been known to become violent in such situations.

Despite plentiful indicators of problems linked to poor frontal lobe function, and despite the close similarity in behaviour with frontal lobe lesion patients, no holes in the frontal lobes have ever been found in autism. There are no visible anatomical abnormalities. But the poor functioning of the frontal lobes could be due to a fault elsewhere, or a fault in connectivity with other brain regions. Investigations are in progress to find out just how the frontal lobes in autism are working during different tasks, when looked at in the scanner. One thing is clear already: they are not functioning as they should, even though they look healthy enough. They seem to be organized differently.

Problems with the idea

The idea of poor executive function is widely accepted. Further, the difficulties in everyday life are widely acknowledged to be present in most individuals with autism. But there is a major problem. The idea is so broad that it might apply to almost all neurodevelopmental disorders, not just autism.

A link between the five big ideas: a mismatch between top-down and bottom-up processes

This section is about ideas that are still only half-baked. So you need to decide whether you would like to roll up your sleeves and join me in the bakery or whether you'd rather skip to the next chapter.

Top-down and bottom-up. I like these terms and use them a lot. I think they capture something very important about how the mind/brain functions. Both these processes are necessary to perceive the world around us and above all to make sense of our perception. Here is a very simplified version of what might be happening:

Let's imagine the brain is divided into two systems. One system is geared to delivering the goods gathered from the outside world, and the other system is geared to controlling what to do next. Roughly speaking, the back of the brain is taken up by delivery processes, while the controlling system is in the front. The delivery system works bottom-up, the control system top-down. Both do a job but they must work together. Now, let's assume that in autism they do not. The proposal is that the bottom-up system is working very well, allowing superior delivery of information and superior performance on any tasks that do not involve the control system but the control system is not working well. This could be true for all of the five big ideas.

When I presented this idea at a conference, a man with Asperger syndrome came up and said he would write to me. His message was: 'Experience has told me that I should never try to understand anything. It works for neurotypicals, but you need top-down thinking to make it work. Analysis and calculation works better for us.' He had after all understood me: he likened top-down control to understanding and bottom-up delivery to analysis and calculation.

What is so important about the top-down system? There is now much evidence from the neuroscience of perception that the brain works by top-down modulation on information that enters the brain bottom-up. Not all information that enters the brain is of equal value. The top-down control system has to sort the good from the bad. It has to convey this to the delivery system. It sends signals that result in useful information being enhanced, and useless information being suppressed. One of the ways by which the top-down system controls the delivery system is through its prior expectations. These are strongly shaped by culture and our social relationships to other people. This brings in the first three big ideas.

The cook and the diner

Imagine a very choosy diner seated upstairs in the dining room, and an extremely busy cook who is doing a lot of work in the kitchen downstairs. Much of the food that the cook offers up is refused, and only choice morsels are deemed worthy of ingestion. The diner has certain preferences and naturally wishes to influence the cook to use only his favourite ingredients. He lets it be known that he is always happy to eat fresh white asparagus of the best quality. The cook, on the other hand, needs to work with the ingredients the market provides.

How does the diner communicate with the cook? By a waiter, of course. The waiter has a hard job. He has to convey to the cook the diner's extravagant orders. He also has to convey to the diner something of the reality of what is going on in the kitchen. The waiter tries to make the diner and the cook work together. He hopes that at least sometimes the diner's preferences will match the cook's speciality of the day.

The waiter has to juggle with two kinds of attention, one that is typical of the cook and one that is typical of the diner. The cook's attention arises entirely from the goods that he secures on the market. For instance, when he goes to market he will be irresistibly attracted by baskets of juicy strawberries. They will grab his attention no matter what. However, there are always many tempting ingredients that capture the cook's fancy. They are then automatically prepared the way they should be: chopped, diced, peeled, steamed, baked, boiled, or fried.

The diner's attention on the other hand, arises from the inside. He never goes to market, but he uses his memory and knowledge he gets from other diners to demand special and often novel food.

Here is an example. Another diner phones our diner and entices him to order duck eggs that are all the rage. The waiter has to spring into action and tell the cook. When the diner wants a duck egg omelette, the cook must stop using chicken eggs and spy out duck eggs.

Sometimes both are working really well together. When the cook delivers the desired omelette, the diner's enjoyment is great. Sometimes top-down attention can be in competition with bottom-up attention. The diner shouts for asparagus while the cook is preoccupied with quelling a kitchen fire. In this case the diner will not get what he desires. However, he may now order a more efficient fire extinguisher.

This parable is meant to illustrate the interplay between the brain's control and delivery systems. Neither is more important than the other. As the last example showed, the controlling system cannot override the emergency in the delivery system. However, it can take action to prevent a recurrence of the emergency. My proposal is that in autism the interplay between these two brain systems does not function well. Is this the fault of an indifferent diner, an overzealous cook, or a confused waiter? It could be any one, but personally, I tend to blame the diner.

Top-down modulation

What happens in the brain during top-down control of visual perception? A brain-imaging experiment gives some clues. In this experiment people were told in advance where to direct their attention on a screen. On the screen pairs of pictures flashed up for a split second. Importantly, the subjects could only just see them and only when they were told in advance where to look. Now the pictures were either faces or houses. This was a clever choice because the brain regions that are active when watching houses and faces are in different places. This is known from other experiments. In this experiment, when houses or faces were shown, these brain regions were indeed active too. What is more, they were more active when attention had been directed—by the experimenter's instruction—to the location where they appeared moments later. In other words, top-down attention enhances brain activity. Autistic people were scanned with exactly the same task. They showed much less enhanced activation. This is direct evidence for a lack of top-down modulation at the level of the brain in autism.

The person who has difficulty modulating attention is prone to being grabbed by external stimuli. At the same time they find it difficult to tear their attention away again. Perhaps this is why Joe eats the same food all the time; why Edward's interests are narrow and restricted; and why David has a superb but literal memory.

The absent diner

This is a rather risky idea—and I only include it because I am hoping to find an answer for the question: What is the top in top-down? My short answer at the moment is that the top in top-down is the Self. This Self is in fact the diner I have conjured up previously. The diner has certain preferences and expectations and constantly influences what is served up to him from the kitchen. So the Self has preferences and influences how the brain processes information. The diner selects what food he wishes to try. The Self decides what is of interest and what is not. An absent Self is one way to characterize the mismatch between bottom-up and top-down processing.

If there was an absent diner, then one would expect that the cook, unhampered by quirky demands from the top, would be able to produce the most gorgeous meals entirely from the ingredients to hand, and entirely doing what he is best at, by using his special skills of chopping, dicing, mashing, steaming, baking, frying. This would be one way to understand savant skills.

But isn't there a problem? What about Joe's insistence on eating exactly the same food? Does this not suggest a very strong Self? Or, in the metaphor, a diner with strongly set prior expectations? I don't think so. After all as described by Michael Blastland, there was no reasoning with Joe about this expectation. The response was impenetrably rigid. To me this suggests simple association learning or instrumental conditioning. Here the top of the command chain is an isolated but engrained response to a stimulus that has been rewarding in the past. This is the cook going it alone, doing the thing he is good at. But to no purpose because there is no diner at the top.

Here we need to recall another feature of the diner, his social interest and capacity to communicate with other diners. He does not merely make a wilful decision of what he wants to eat, but he is influenced by what other diners are eating, indeed by what is currently fashionable. We could imagine not so much an absent diner but a diner who doesn't communicate with other diners.

Some preliminary conclusions

In this chapter the non-social features of autism were in the spotlight. These include both strengths and weaknesses. The fourth idea, called weak central coherence, allowed us to celebrate the strengths of autistic people and give credit to their special talents. The fifth idea, often referred to as executive dysfunction, is concerned with their countless difficulties in managing everyday life.

I have contrasted strengths in one system of the brain—to do with delivery of information, with weaknesses in another system—to do with control of information. The evidence suggests that there is a weakness in the control system of the brain, but strength in the delivery system.

In the last part of this chapter, I have tried to speculate about a mismatch between top-down and bottom-up processes. But many questions remain open. Why are autistic people different in just the way they are? Why don't they share the social and physical world of other people? I have put the blame on the top-down controlling system of the brain, and have put the blame on an absent Self, or at least a Self that lacks normal interaction with other social beings.

Will there eventually be a satisfying formulation of the idea to explain the specifically autistic tendencies of getting stuck and lacking flexibility? Perhaps. Can the notion of the absent Self capture the autism-characteristic mismatch between top-down control and bottom-up delivery? Just possibly.

Chapter 7
From theory to practice

A trick with three boxes

In her exploration of autism, Diane surveyed many facts, saw many faces of autism, and learned about psychological experiments that have tried to penetrate deeply into the mind of the person with autism. What does it all add up to? Is there a grand unified theory? Unfortunately not. Autistic disorders are far too heterogeneous and too complex for a single satisfying account.

Nevertheless, Diane wanted to have a picture to give shape to what she has learned. She was still fascinated and now contemplated whether she should start doing some research on autism herself. With her background in natural sciences she is well equipped to pick up the necessary techniques of neuroscience. Putting together what she now knows seems a good idea. She could then see what is missing and what work needs to be done to obtain a more complete account of autism in the future.

Here is a little help. First, Diane has to tidy up the many different bits of knowledge that she has. This tidying is helped enormously by a simple trick: put different bits of knowledge into three different boxes. Let's call them *biology, mind, behaviour*. Each box is for a particular type of knowledge: in the *biology* box is knowledge gathered so far about the brain and genes; in the *mind* box are insights gained from experimental studies about the mind; and in the *behaviour* box are well-established facts about behaviour. In each box she can put lists with things she knows.

The remarkable thing that comes out of this tidying operation is that the *mind* box is the essential link between the other two. In the box for *behaviour* Diane has a list of the signs and symptoms of autism in their various and changing forms. Chapters 1 and 2 contain a lot of these facts. In the box for *biology*, she has a list of facts, some of which are presented in Chapters 3 and 4.

The *mind* box is filled with ideas that have been discussed in the last two chapters. Here we put ideas rather than facts and that is alright. The ideas are all testable and they are not taken out of the blue. They are my personal best bets for standing the test of time, and they are all backed by sound experimental studies. There are strong hints to the neural underpinnings of these features—but only hints. Diane is itching to do some of this work herself.

What we find in the biology box

For the causes of autism Diane has made a long list of factors: developmental instability, genetic predispositions, mutations, environmental risk factors, chance and accidents. These different possibilities are not exclusive and not necessarily separate from each other. Instead they may combine to lead to the large variety of disorders on the autism spectrum. As yet it seems difficult to sort out different causes at the genetic level. Different causes may affect a final common pathway, which causes similar brain-mind abnormalities and similar signs and symptoms.

Very little is as yet known about the brain in autism. Children with autism have larger brains; not at birth, but a rapid increase can be observed after the first year of life, followed by a levelling off at around eight years or so. This fact could be related to waxing and waning of neural connections: a massive proliferation of neural connections followed by savage pruning. A disturbance in these highly complex and dynamic processes might be the final common pathway of many different causes.

What we find in the behaviour box

Diane recalls that autism is currently identified by behaviour. Here she lists the core features of autism and also other features that are common, such as hypersensitivity and echoing of speech. Behavioural features are problematic because they change with age, with ability, with many factors causing differences that are not part of the underlying condition. There are no unique sets of behaviours, which will unequivocally identify autism. Two children whose autism is caused by the same biological factor may nevertheless appear different from each other. Each individual will show a different pattern of behaviour. It all depends on many factors, their own inner resources, their education, and the support they get from the outside. It is satisfying to know that a supportive educational environment can have a massive influence. It can even mask existing problems. How exactly do these influences operate? We still don't know.

What we find in the mind box

Obviously the five big ideas go into the mind box. These ideas can pull together bits and pieces lodged in the behavioural box that at first seemed unrelated. Diane knows straightaway that there would be more such ideas if she searched further. But five is a good start. The mind box would be useful as a temporary dumping ground for all the ideas and theories she would hear about autism in the future, and would invent herself. Importantly, there has to be some vetting and a need for strict testing once they are admitted. The plausible idea of a lack of social drive, the strange idea of mentalizing, and the novel idea of the broken mirror all make sense of different aspects of the hallmark of autism: the lack of reciprocal social interaction. The theory of weak central coherence tries to explain savant skills and the different way of seeing the world in general. The theory of poor executive function tries to explain all the daily difficulties in autism. All in all, the five big ideas together make sense of many of the puzzling phenomena that are thrown up by autism. Furthermore, they provide clues about the underlying neural mechanisms that might have gone wrong.

How the boxes might fit together

It is frustrating that there is no answer yet to what causes autism. There are many different risk factors, genetic and environmental. The effect of these causes is on the mind as much as it is on the brain. There might be a common pathway in the brain/mind that is ultimately affected. This would mean something quite important. Even if autism is extremely variable as far as its causes and as far as the resulting behaviour patterns are concerned, there is some common denominator. This is a cognitive phenotype. Perhaps there are more than one common pathway and more than one cognitive phenotype. This would be the case if distinct subgroups on the autism spectrum could be identified.

What if each of the five big ideas defined a cognitive phenotype? Basically you can think of a cognitive phenotype as encapsulating one of the big ideas. Perhaps this division would make the search for the causes of autism simpler. Could there be five types of autism? Possibly. But there is another possibility. The faults suggested by the five big ideas could be all mixed together like ingredients in a cake. The ingredients might be added in different quantities, and some might be optional. It is possible to imagine that different mixes would represent different points on the autism spectrum.

Let's take the example of mentalizing again. Could a mentalizing fault define a subgroup of the autism spectrum? What types of *autistic* behaviour would this explain? It could explain the core feature of an inability to engage in truly reciprocal social interaction and communication. This encompasses a big range of behaviours, which we have touched on in earlier chapters. It would fit each of our three example cases, even though David, Gary, and Edward are at very different points of the autism spectrum.

How would you identify a mentalizing fault in each case when their abilities are so varied, when the education and support they received is so vastly different? You would need a large battery of tests. And this does not exist yet. These tests have to give a choice of the right level of difficulty; they have to be reliable and they have to be ultimately linked with real-life behaviour. In principle, individual cases could be assessed using brain imaging. Given that the brain's mentalizing system has been isolated, abnormal function should be visible in this system. Existing results suggest that there should be weaker connections between the components of the system.

Let's take another example. Do David, Gary, and Edward show a cognitive phenotype of weak central coherence? This phenotype represents individuals who by preference will focus attention on details and cannot easily be distracted away. A battery of tests is again needed—tests of the right difficulty level, reliability, and validity. These would probably include tests of attention and tests of intelligence. One of the aims of the weak central coherence idea is after all to explain an uneven pattern of intelligence. We might suspect that Gary would not have this phenotype—he did not have outstanding abilities or narrow interests—but David probably would. He excelled at jigsaw puzzles, for instance. In Edward's case we might also find a big difference between his best and worst performance. Tests of signature brain activation patterns are still in the future. One might expect that they would show misconnections. This might mean too few connections between distant brain regions and too many between nearby regions. A traffic analogy comes to mind: no big highways, but a multitude of small local roads.

For Diane the boxes are beginning to fit together. Misconnections might be the reason that there is a lack of mentalizing, a lack of social drive, a broken mirror system, weak central coherence, and trouble with top-down control.

Connections and misconnections in the brain

Let's assume that in the autistic brain the wires are crossed, literally. For instance, normally, when people read minds, parts of the brain immediately get active and work in synchrony. In autism it looks as if this is not the case. Perhaps the connections between the mind-reading parts of the brain are weak precisely because there are too few of the big highway connections between these relatively distant regions, some of which are in the middle of the brain, some on the sides, and some in the back.

Autism is a neurodevelopmental disorder, which appears to be due to a disorganization of brain development. This now makes sense to Diane. But she needs another step in the argument. The disorganization might be due to lack of pruning of particular neural connections. She has to address one other issue: Why is autism apparent only from the second year of life? She asks what kinds of brain connections proliferate in the second year of life. I can only give a guess, but it could plausibly be the connections in the controlling system. From work on the visual part of the brain in animals we know that the bottom-up connections of the delivery system of the brain are ready and waiting well before the top-down connections of the controlling system are mature.

Let's assume it is the top-down connections that first proliferate and then have to be pruned. It could be that in autism precisely these connections are not cut back as quickly as they should be. If so, this would explain three things in one fell swoop: the excellent perceptual abilities of a great delivery system; the limited modulation abilities of a stalled control system, and the start of autistic symptoms in the second year. Just possibly it would also explain the bulge in brain size in autism after the first year of life.

Diane decides that a good research project would be to try and engineer a misconnected brain, for example in a mouse. How would it function? How would she test the mouse? It should have an uneven pattern of abilities. It should be able to do some tasks well, others not so well, especially tasks that need top-down control, and those that need a refined social sense.

I am delighted that Diane has decided to tackle this problem. With the right sorts of task it should be possible to show that there are systems in the brain that normally work together, but are more weakly connected in the autistic brain. I believe that in the end something has to be identified as the top in top-down, and this is what has to take the responsibility for the control. I myself have wondered whether this is a form of the Self. Is this Self absent in autism? Does this reveal a deeper meaning of the word for autism, which is after all derived from the Greek word for Self, *autos*? I cannot give an answer. However, I am looking forward with hope and fascination to the next wave of experimental investigations.

Tensions in the concept of the autism spectrum

In the course of writing this book I have been acutely aware of a tension in using examples sometimes of severe and classic cases of autism and sometimes very high-functioning cases and Asperger syndrome. There is also a gulf between the examples taken from cases of children and of adults. The anecdotes about what it feels like to be autistic all come from high-functioning adults. There is a danger therefore that the view of autism spectrum disorders is heavily weighted towards this part of the spectrum. It is not necessarily correct to call it the mild part, because these people have disabilities. They are sometimes rather thinly covered up by compensatory efforts. On the other hand, their autistic features are mild compared to the classic cases.

In the research I have reported, experiments often rely on participants with normal or high intelligence because the techniques and tasks are very demanding. These have revealed fascinating results and I make no apology for drawing on them extensively. When I remember classic cases that I know, then it seems to me that all the five big ideas are relevant to explain their behaviour, and they seem to apply simultaneously. This is not the case when I survey the high-functioning cases. Here I have the feeling that in individual cases some but not necessarily all of the big ideas are needed to explain their difficulties.

All this makes me think that it would be a good idea in future research to ask separate questions about severe autism, usually accompanied by intellectual impairment and milder forms of autism usually without intellectual impairment. It may not be possible to generalize research findings from one group to the other. The following section addresses some of the more practical questions about autism, and here it is obvious that it is necessary to treat these subgroups separately. Let's start with the highly intelligent.

Throughout this book we have had numerous occasions to look at examples of exceptional people, who have an autistic condition and who can tell us about their experiences. Temple Grandin is such a person. She has achieved accolades as a writer, presenter, and a researcher of animal behaviour. Temple Grandin's website illustrates her many astonishing talents. She can articulate what it means to have high-functioning autism and she highlights certain advantages of the thinking style, which in her own case, she describes as visual thinking. She is content to be on her own and demonstrates that it is possible to live a fulfilled life without the ability to engage in reciprocal communication. Nor is Temple Grandin the only person with autism who has written about her life, her interests, and inner experience. There are many books now by highly talented writers who reveal from a first-person point of view what it is like to have autism.

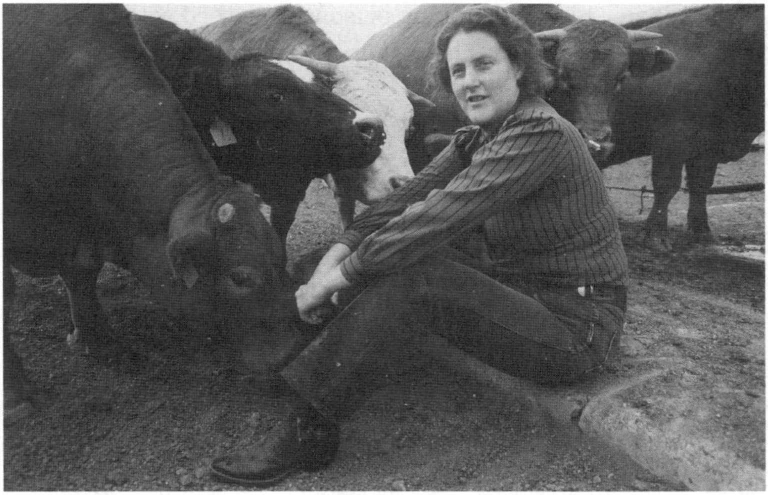

19. Temple Grandin is a spokesperson for able people with autism. She has written books on what it is like to be autistic. She designs livestock equipment and has a special affinity for animals. She wrote about this in her book, *Animals in Translation: Using the Mysteries of Autism to Decode Animal Behavior* (New York: Scribner, 2005)

If you met someone like Temple Grandin

This would be a little bit like meeting a pop star. It is more likely that you would run into someone like Edward, whose case we have looked at repeatedly. You may *not* immediately notice that Edward is 'different'. Nevertheless, for Edward to look and act normal is a tremendous effort. It may surprise you that he is very anxious, even panic stricken while you merely chat inconsequentially. In Edward's mind, anything might happen. You might suddenly turn hostile; you may suddenly make an unreasonable demand. One can make allowances for this by listening patiently and making reassuring remarks. As a rule it pays to be direct and firm. Edward would probably not take polite hints from you as signals to stop talking about bird's eggs. With luck, Edward will find a job in academia. He may even make a great discovery in a field of mathematics.

Beware. Some high-functioning persons diagnosed with an autistic condition may yet turn out not to belong to the autism spectrum but to have some other personality problem. Of course they may convince you that they have Asperger syndrome. But you can see the danger of circularity. A hard look at the boundaries of the autism spectrum will be necessary to get out of this circle.

If you met someone with autism and intellectual disabilities

Very different things would strike you when meeting Sylvia at age 40. You would know straight away that she has 'special needs'. Sylvia was a classically autistic girl who showed aloofness and insistence on sameness. She had talents as well as difficulties. She did well at a specialist school, but unfortunately, during adolescence her behaviour problems increased. She also developed epilepsy. As she became physically strong, her frustration at not understanding things often resulted in breaking things and hurting others and herself. She now needs constant supervision. Her family have no time for the notion that autism is just a difference and not a disorder. They feel this claim as cruel mockery. There is no doubt that autism has blighted Sylvia's life. But should we grieve for her and bemoan her fate? Not necessarily. Sylvia is only dimly aware of her own problems, and is as happy as anyone else who can live in a loving environment.

What about Gary? You would certainly know that there is something odd about him. You might be put off by his unkempt looks and uncouth behaviour. When you meet him, you would probably think he is a tramp. He often grumbles about not being given a fair chance, but actually, he is quite content as long as he is left in peace. Since joining the Asperger support group he has found people he feels comfortable with and counts as friends. He has even found a girlfriend among them. He may never find employment, and when he is no longer able to live at home, he will depend on social services for housing and support.

What does it cost to have an autism spectrum disorder?

Health economists make it their business to find out just how much it costs to take care of a person with an autism spectrum condition over a lifetime. In the case of Great Britain such estimates are £2.9 million for a high-functioning person with autism and £4.7 million for a low-functioning person—over a lifetime. Most of the funding currently goes on living support. However, there is less than ideal provision in many cases. The social services and special education services are chronically short of funds and could easily use more to enhance and improve their work.

It is one thing to estimate the financial burden, but the human costs are another, and cannot be estimated at all. Clearly, it is imperative to ameliorate the burden of autism.

Education and remediation

There are plenty of practical guides to educating the high-functioning and the low-functioning child respectively. Fortunately, there are effective educational programmes for children with severe autism. I have already mentioned Applied Behavioural Analysis (ABA). Here appropriate skills and behaviours are taught through learning theory principles. There is music therapy and art therapy, which are beneficial in their own right. Speech therapy can help enormously to promote articulation and the use of language. Therapies are never as easy as they sound and trained therapists are needed. A combination of several techniques is often the right answer. A gifted and committed teacher or parent makes all the difference, which is another way of saying that we don't really know what the magic ingredient is.

Some of the techniques used involve quite intense social affective interactions and games. For example, the kind of larger than life interactions enhanced by modulated voices and facial expressions that mothers use with babies. For older children and adolescents, social skills training is popular and effective. Attractive materials are available, for instance cartoons and films presenting emotional expressions in a very clear form.

One example is *Thomas the Tank Engine*, a much loved children's book, which seems to be a particular favourite with autistic children. Parents believe that the clear facial expressions on the little railway engines and the simple stories of social interactions,

20. W. V. Awdry wrote the Railway series of books for children. *Thomas the Tank Engine* appeared first in 1946 and continues to enjoy great popularity. Autistic children are attracted to the pictures of railway engines with their big personalities and their expressive faces, and can learn about social signals through the stories

illustrating, for instance, cooperation, competition, pride, anxiety, and jealousy, are appealing enough to work as teaching aids. 'The names of the engines were the first words he used before Mum and Dad', was reported by more than one set of parents.

The Cambridge Autism Research Centre, whose website is easy to access, uses the idea of little engines, called Transporters. These heroes of tailor-made stories act as teaching aids for social skills and social signals. They show clear, simplified expressions of emotions. It is the simplicity of design and storyline that appears to enhance learning and make it enjoyable.

What kind of educational and social provisions are needed?

Deciding about education, employment, and living accommodation in later life are not one-off decisions. In discussions about the needs and rights of individuals with autism, people often get very confused because the autism spectrum is so wide. It is not possible to make general provisions that catch all. The diversity of services that are needed is enormous.

This is true for education as well. Discussions about special needs schools and integrated schooling are never ending. Parents may have strong preferences for their child to be placed in a mainstream school, thinking that this is the place where—driven by the sheer need to get along with other children—their child would be able to adapt and learn social skills. If only this were so! Instead, most children with autism seem to benefit from being taught by a specialist teacher in the calm and highly structured environment of a special unit or special school. But this is not an opinion shared by all, and the debate will continue. There are so many shades of autism that it seems sensible to make individual plans for individual children.

Medical treatments

Medical treatments for autism do not exist. However, secondary symptoms, for example, epilepsy, high anxiety, or depression, are amenable to being improved by medication. In autistic conditions, just as in typical development, it is necessary to be vigilant about all sorts of medical conditions. Many of these seem to occur unusually often in children with autism, for instance, gastric inflammation, or allergic reactions. Many of these are treatable.

If a child has gastric inflammation but does not know how to communicate this, then this child might well show a range of behaviour problems, such as biting and screaming. If the inflammation was treated with the appropriate medication, then the child would be much calmer and happier, even though the underlying problem in communication has not gone away.

Dietary interventions have their passionate proponents. Bad reactions to food allergies may well have an impact on behaviour, and taking account of these allergies makes sense. However, only some autistic children are likely to suffer from such allergies.

Charlatans

As long as there is a demand for a cure for autism, there will be people who say they can supply a cure. We certainly have no indication that autism is a disease like tuberculosis that can be cured thanks to modern pharmaceuticals. As we discussed in Chapter 4, autism is a largely genetically-based condition, with a rainbow of different facets of manifestations in behaviour. The condition is not always a disorder and not always a burden. Clearly it is absurd to wish for a cure in these cases. It is not absurd to wish for amelioration or prevention in those cases where disabilities dominate the picture. As yet, we have no proper knowledge of how to do this. Anyone who promises a short-cut, be it through taking a particular dietary supplement or other regime, should be suspected of being a charlatan. Luckily, there are websites that warn of potentially dangerous and unproven therapies.

One thing is worth knowing if you are a parent, carer, or teacher. Development is a strong force. Improvements over time, in behaviour, in social skills, and in language, are only to be expected. This is true also for the child with autism. Nothing special has to happen for these improvements to occur, over and above a typical level of care and support. This means that special interventions have to be measured against expected improvements. It is likely that educational programmes deliver significant improvements over and above these expected improvements. However, evaluating these programmes is extremely difficult. There is as yet only good practice rather than a consensus on optimal practice.

Stress

It is quite obvious that caring for a child who is unable to communicate and engage in reciprocal communication, who has rigid behaviour patterns and obsessive tendencies, is a heavy burden to bear for any family. Even in families who have vast material resources and a community network that provides services for such a child, it remains a hard task. Spare a thought also for the siblings of the child with autism.

Parents will thank you for not criticizing their methods of keeping control of tense situations. Be sympathetic when you see a family struggling to make a journey by plane, and their autistic child obsessively asks to have a drink. Yes, they probably have thought of giving him a drink! And no, they are not callous or inept. No doubt they have found out by experience that they must ignore the repeated request.

The main stress on the family is not 'what other people think'. One can get immune to raised eyebrows and know-better suggestions.

The main stress is all to do with the many open questions about autism. How frustrating it is not to know what causes the condition. If we knew, I believe parents' attitudes would change from bewilderment to a better ability to cope and to an increased chance of acceptance. Many can achieve acceptance and many gain a positive outlook, even happiness. But this is not the norm.

The effect of stress on the individual with autism is probably much worse than on healthy people. If it can be avoided, then things can go nicely in well-worked-out routines. Conversely, if there is a sudden deterioration of behaviour, look for the stress that might have caused it. So the best possible practical advice for those who are in daily contact with an autistic person is often just this: try and find out what the stressors are and remove them. They may not be obvious. For example, it may simply be an unstructured situation, as when having to make a decision of what to eat.

You don't need to be afraid of people with autism. They are different, but just like Christopher, the hero of Mark Haddon's novel, they often try very hard to be like everybody else. They might overdo it, and they may get on other people's nerves, for example, by asking strange questions at an awkward time. It is possible to cope with this better if you have gained some basic knowledge and understanding from basic research. Rather than looking for specific advice of what to say or do, which never fits the individual or the exact situation, you can formulate and think through a question yourself.

The message in this book is that scientific research has already answered some of the puzzling questions about autism and in the future will provide answers to the many questions that are still open. To decide about the proper education and care of people with autism there is no short-cut. It is essential that research is done at a very basic level, especially at the level of brain and mind.

Things we need to know more about

The puzzle of autism still beckons to be solved. In this book I have indicated black spots of ignorance in many places. Above all we need to know more about how the mind/brain works. For instance, what happens in the brain when we experience empathy, when we make eye contact, when we recognize faces, in short, when we engage in social communication with another person? We need to know more about mechanisms in the mind/brain that enable us to become aware of ourselves and of our relationship with others. Perhaps, most tantalizing of all, we need to find the secret of savant talents.

However, we can also look at these black spots of ignorance as white spots on an as-yet-unexplored continent. Explorers of all kinds, especially those who can combine psychological experiments and techniques of neuroscience, and can work hand in hand with cell biologists and geneticists, will fill in the map and will come back with answers that promise rich rewards. These answers will not only make us able to understand people with autism better, they will make us understand why all of us are who we are.

My advice to Diane is that she should not be afraid to create other big ideas and take a hard and critical look at those that are presented in this book. There is no better way to push back the frontiers of knowledge than by trying out ideas that seem a little outrageous at first—so long as they can be tested experimentally.

Specialist references

See also references cited in the captions to Figures.

On prevalence

Baird, G., Simonoff, E., Pickles, A., Chandler, S., Loucas, T., Meldrum, D., Charman, T. (2006) Prevalence of disorders of the autism spectrum in a population cohort of children in South Thames: the Special Needs and Autism Project (SNAP). *Lancet*, **368(9531)**: 210–15.

Baron-Cohen, S., Wheelwright, S., Skinner, R., Martin, J., and Clubley, E. (2001) The autism spectrum quotient (AQ): evidence from Asperger syndrome/high-functioning autism, males and females, scientists and mathematicians. *Journal of Autism and Developmental Disorders*, **31**: 5–17.

Wing, L., and Potter, D. (2002) The epidemiology of autistic spectrum disorders: is the prevalence rising? *Mental Retardation and Developmental Disabilities Research Reviews*, **8(3)**: 151–61.

On causes

Bauman, M. L., and Kemper, T. L., eds. (1994) *The Neurobiology of Autism*. Baltimore: Johns Hopkins University Press.

Courchesne, E. (2004) Brain development in autism: early overgrowth followed by premature arrest of growth. *Mental Retardation and Developmental Disability Research Reviews* **10(2)**: 106–11.

Ellman, D., and Bedford, H. (2007) MMR: where are we now? *Archives of Disease in Childhood*, **92**: 1055–7.

Geschwind, D., and Levitt, P. (2007) Autism spectrum disorders: developmental disconnection syndromes. *Current Opinion in Neurobiology*, **17(1)**: 103–11.

Gillberg, C. and Coleman, M. (2000) *The Biology of the autistic syndromes* 3rd ed. London: Mac Keith Press.

Losh, M. and Piven, J. (2007) Social cognition and the broad autism phenotype: identifying genetically meaningful phenotypes. *Journal of Child Psychology and Psychiatry*, **48(1)**: 105–12.

Minshew, N.J. and Williams D.L. (2007) The new neurobiology of autism: cortex, connectivity, and neuronal organization. *Archives of Neurology*, **64(7)**: 945–50.

Persico, A. M., and Bourgeron, T. (2006) Searching for ways out of the autism maze: genetic, epigenetic and environmental clues. *Trends in Neuroscience*, **29(7)**: 349–58.

Rutter, M. (2006) *Genes and Behavior: Nature-Nurture Interplay Explained.* Oxford: Blackwell.

Yeo, R. A., Gangestad, S. W., and Thoma, R. J. (2007) Developmental instability and individual variation in brain development: implications for the origin of neurodevelopmental disorders. *Current Directions in Psychological Science*, **16**: 245–9.

On impairments of social interaction

Baron-Cohen, S., Tager-Flusberg, H., and Cohen, D., eds. (2000) *Understanding Other Minds: Perspectives from Developmental Cognitive Neuroscience.* Oxford: Oxford University Press.

Dapretto, M., Davies, M. S., Pfeifer, J. J., Scott, A. A., Sigman, M., Bookheimer, S. Y. *et al.* (2006) Understanding emotions in others: mirror neuron dysfunction in children with autism spectrum disorders. *Nature Neuroscience*, **9(1)**: 28–30.

Dawson, G., Meltzoff, A. N., Osterling, J., Rinaldi, J., and Brown, E. (1998) Children with autism fail to orient to naturally occurring social stimuli. *Journal of Autism and Developmental Disorders*, **28(6)**: 479–85.

Hirschfeld, L., Bartmess, E., White, S., and Frith, U. (2007). Can autistic children predict behavior by social stereotypes? *Current Biology*, **17(12)**: R451–2.

Mundy, P., and Newell, L. (2007) Attention, joint attention and social cognition. *Current Directions in Psychological Science*, **16(5)**: 269–74.

Pelphrey, K., Morris, J. P., McCarthy, G. (2005) The neurological basis of eye gaze processing deficits in autism. *Brain*, **128** (Pt 5): 1038–48.

Rizzolatti, G., Fogassi, L., Gallese, V. (2006) Mirrors of the mind. *Scientific American*, **295(5)**: 54–61.

Rogers, S., and Williams J. H. G., eds. (2006) *Imitation and the Social Mind: Typical Development and Autism*. New York: Guilford Press.

On non-social features

Bird, G., Catmur, C., Silani, G., Frith, C., Frith, U. (2006) Attention does not modulate neural responses to social stimuli in autism spectrum disorders. *Neuroimage*, **31(4)**: 1614–24.

Gilbert S.J., Bird G., Brindley R., Frith C.D. and Burgess P.W. (2008) Atypical recruitment of medial prefrontal cortex in autism spectrum disorders: An fMRI study of two executive function tasks, *Neuropsychologia*, **46(9)**: 2281-91.

Happé, F., and Frith, U. (2006) The weak central coherence account: detail focused cognitive style in autistic spectrum disorders. *Journal of Autism and Developmental Disorders*, **36**: 5–25.

Heaton, P., Williams, K., Cummins, O., and Happé, F. (2007) Autism and pitch processing splinter skills: a group and subgroup analysis. *Autism*, 12: 203–19.

Hermelin, B. (2001) *Bright Splinters of the Mind: A Personal Story of Research with Autistic Savants*. London: Jessica Kingsley.

Hill, E.L. (2004) Executive dysfunction in autism. *Trends in Cognitive Sciences*, **8(1)**: 26–32.

Mann T.A. and Walker P. (2003) Autism and a deficit in broadening the spread of visual attention, *Journal of Child Psychology and Psychiatry*, **44(2)**: 274–84.

Mottron, L., Dawson, M., Soulieres, I., Hubert, B., and Burack, J. (2006) Enhanced perceptual functioning in autism: an update, and eight principles of autistic perception. *Journal of Autism and Developmental Disorders*, **36(1)**: 27–43.

Further reading

Classic readings

Asperger, H. (1944) Die 'autistischen Psychopathen', in *Kindesalter*, trans. U. Frith in U. Frith, ed. (1991) *Autism and Asperger Syndrome*. Cambridge: Cambridge University Press.

Kanner, L. (1943) Autistic disturbances of affective contact, *Nervous Child*, **2**: 217–50.

Introductions

Frith, U. (2003) *Autism: Explaining the Enigma*. Oxford: Blackwell.

Medical Research Council UK (2001) *Autism: Research Review*, MRC website.

Sigman, M., and Capps, L. (1997) *Children with Autism: A Developmental Perspective*. Cambridge, Mass.: Harvard University Press.

Houston, R., and Frith, U. (2002) *Autism in History*. Oxford: Blackwell.

Morton, J. (2004) *Understanding Developmental Disorders: A Cognitive Modelling Approach*. Oxford: Blackwell.

Edited volumes presenting research

Charman, T., and Stone, W., eds. (2006) *Social and Communication Development in Autism Spectrum Disorders: Early Identification, Diagnosis, and Intervention*. New York: Guilford Press.

Frith, U., and Hill, E., eds. (2003) *Autism: Brain and Mind*, Oxford: Oxford University Press.
McGregor, E., Nunez, M., Cebula, K., and Gomez, J. C. *et al.*, eds. (2008) *Autism: An Integrated View from Neurocognitive, Clinical and Intervention Research.* Oxford: Wiley-Blackwell.
Volkmar, F. R., Paul, R., Klin, A., and Cohen, D. J., eds. (2005) *Handbook of Autism and Pervasive Developmental Disorders, Diagnosis, Development, Neurobiology, and Behavior*, 3rd edition. Hoboken, NJ: Wiley.

Biographical accounts

Claiborne-Park, C. (1967, 1995) *The Siege.* New York: Little Brown.
Blastland, M. (2006) *Joe: The Only Boy in the World.* London: Profile Books.
Grandin, T. (1996) *Thinking in Pictures: My Life with Autism.* New York: Vintage Books.
Lawson, W. (2000) *Life behind Glass: A Personal Account of Autism Spectrum Disorder.* London: Jessica Kingsley.
Moore, C. (2004) *George and Sam.* London: Penguin.
Sacks, O. (1995) *An Anthropologist on Mars.* New York: Vintage Books.

Guide books

Attwood, T. (2006) *A Complete Guide to Asperger's Syndrome.* London: Jessica Kingsley.
Siegel, B. (2003) *Helping Children with Autism Learn: Treatment Approaches for Parents and Professionals.* Oxford: Oxford University Press.
Wing. L. (1997) *The Autism Spectrum: A Guide for Parents and Professionals.* London: Constable.

“牛津通识读本”已出书目

古典哲学的趣味
人生的意义
文学理论入门
大众经济学
历史之源
设计，无处不在
生活中的心理学
政治的历史与边界
哲学的思与惑
资本主义
美国总统制
海德格尔
我们时代的伦理学
卡夫卡是谁
考古学的过去与未来
天文学简史
社会学的意识
康德
尼采
亚里士多德的世界
西方艺术新论
全球化面面观
简明逻辑学
法哲学：价值与事实
政治哲学与幸福根基
选择理论
后殖民主义与世界格局

福柯
缤纷的语言学
达达和超现实主义
佛学概论
维特根斯坦与哲学
科学哲学
印度哲学祛魅
克尔凯郭尔
科学革命
广告
数学
叔本华
笛卡尔
基督教神学
犹太人与犹太教
现代日本
罗兰·巴特
马基雅维里
全球经济史
进化
性存在
量子理论
牛顿新传
国际移民
哈贝马斯
医学伦理
黑格尔

地球
记忆
法律
中国文学
托克维尔
休谟
分子
法国大革命
民族主义
科幻作品
罗素
美国政党与选举
美国最高法院
纪录片
大萧条与罗斯福新政
领导力
无神论
罗马共和国
美国国会
民主
英格兰文学
现代主义
网络
自闭症
德里达
浪漫主义
批判理论

德国文学
戏剧
腐败
医事法
癌症
植物
法语文学
微观经济学
湖泊
拜占庭
司法心理学
发展
农业
特洛伊战争
巴比伦尼亚
河流
战争与技术
品牌学

儿童心理学
时装
现代拉丁美洲文学
卢梭
隐私
电影音乐
抑郁症
传染病
希腊化时代
知识
环境伦理学
美国革命
元素周期表
人口学
社会心理学
动物
项目管理
美学

电影
俄罗斯文学
古典文学
大数据
洛克
幸福
免疫系统
银行学
景观设计学
神圣罗马帝国
大流行病
亚历山大大帝
气候
第二次世界大战
中世纪
工业革命
传记